Evidence Synthesis and Meta-Analysis for Drug Safety

Report of CIOMS Working Group X

Council for International Organizations of Medical Sciences (CIOMS)

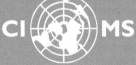

Geneva 2016

All rights reserved. CIOMS publications may be obtained directly from:

CIOMS, P.O. Box 2100, CH-1211 Geneva 2, Switzerland, tel.: +41 22 791 6497, www.cioms.ch, e-mail: info@cioms.ch.

CIOMS publications are also available through the World Health Organization, WHO Press, 20 Avenue Appia, CH-1211 Geneva 27, Switzerland.

Citations:
CIOMS Working Group X. Evidence Synthesis and Meta-Analysis for Drug Safety: Report of CIOMS Working Group X. Geneva, Switzerland: Council for International Organizations of Medical Sciences (CIOMS), 2016.

The authors alone are responsible for the views expressed in this publication and those views do not necessarily represent the decisions, policies or views of their respective institutions or companies.

This publication uses the World Health Organization's *WHO style guide*, 2nd Edition, 2013 (WHO/KMS/WHP/13.1) for spelling, punctuation, terminology and formatting which combines British and American English conventions.

References in this document retain their unique number throughout the document and at the end of each chapter.

Design and Layout: Paprika (Annecy, France)

ACKNOWLEDGEMENTS

During its many years of existence, one of the roles of the Council for International Organizations of Medical Sciences (CIOMS) has been to take up debatable scientific topics. Evidence synthesis and meta-analysis of safety data is not an exception in this respect. Since the start of this CIOMS Working Group X on Meta-Analysis of Safety Data within the Regulatory System, members have strived to find solutions and harmonized ways of approaching different challenges within this topic, including agreements on definitions and terminology. The very exciting mix of specialized biostatisticians, epidemiologists and medical experts within regulatory drug safety that characterized the CIOMS Working Group X contributed to interesting discussions and additional clarifications.

CIOMS gratefully acknowledges the contributions of the members of the Working Group as well as the generous support from drug and regulatory authorities, industry, and other organizations and institutions which, by providing these experts and resources, facilitated the work that resulted in this publication. Each member participated actively in the discussions, drafting and redrafting of texts and their review, which enabled the Working Group to bring the entire project to a successful conclusion. During the process, new members were invited according to their expertise. CIOMS thanks especially all members who chaired the meetings of the Working Group for their dedication and capable leadership. Each of the meetings had a nominated rapporteur (or rapporteurs), and CIOMS acknowledges their professional contributions.

The Editorial Group, comprising Drs Brenda Crowe, Jesse Berlin, Tarek Hammad, Bert Leufkens and Tongtong Wang, merits special mention and thanks. CIOMS wishes to express special appreciation to Dr Brenda Crowe who, as Editor-in-Chief of the final report, assured the quality of the publication, and to the chapter leads for coordinating teams and drafts. CIOMS and the Working Group are grateful for valuable input received on several points of the report from member Stephen Evans and senior experts outside the Group who during their review made valuable suggestions: Drs Harald Herkner, Peter Lane, Nancy Dreyer and Julian Higgins.

The work has required a number of meetings organized by the CIOMS Secretariat, and contributions from regulatory agencies and pharmaceutical companies that hosted the meetings (see Annex III) are especially acknowledged. At CIOMS Dr Gunilla Sjölin-Forsberg and and the late Dr Juhana E. Idänpään-Heikkilä, Ms Karin Holm, Ms Amanda Owden, and Ms Sue le Roux managed the project. Ms Karin Holm, contributing with technical collaboration support and coordination of the editorial work, merits special thanks.

Geneva, Switzerland, July 2016

Lembit Rägo, MD, PhD
Secretary-General, CIOMS
(2016–present)

Gunilla Sjölin-Forsberg, MD, PhD
Former Secretary-General, CIOMS
(2010-2015)

The late Juhana E. Idänpään-Heikkilä, MD, PhD
Senior Adviser, CIOMS (2006–2015)
Secretary-General, CIOMS (2000–2006)

TABLE OF CONTENTS

LIST OF TABLES AND FIGURES

ACRONYMS

AE	Adverse events
AEMG	Adverse Effects Methods Group
AHRQ	Agency for Healthcare Research and Quality (U.S.)
BEST	Breast cancer Erythropoietin Survival Trial
CHMP	Committee for Medicinal Products for Human Use (EU)
CI	Confidence interval
CIOMS	Council for International Organizations of Medical Sciences (Switzerland)
COPD	Chronic obstructive pulmonary disease
CRF	Case report form
CVD	Cardiovascular disease
EMA	European Medicines Agency
ENCePP	European Network of Centres for Pharmacoepidemiology and Pharmacovigilance
ESA	Erythropoiesis-stimulating agents
EU	European Union
FDA	Food and Drug Administration (U.S.)
ICH	International Council for Harmonisation of Technical Requirements for Registration of Pharmaceuticals for Human Use
IPD	Individual participant-level data
I^2	I-squared
LIL	Law of iterated logarithms
MA	Meta-analysis
MCMC	Markov chain Monte Carlo
MedDRA	Medical Dictionary for Regulatory Activities
MI	Myocardial infarction
MOOSE	Meta-analysis of Observational Studies in Epidemiology
NNT	Number needed to treat
NSAID	Non-steroidal anti-inflammatory drugs
OR	Odds ratio
PBRER	Periodic benefit–risk evaluation report
PRISMA	Preferred Reporting Items for Systematic Reviews and Meta-Analyses
RCT	Randomized controlled clinical trials
RD	Risk difference
RR	Risk ratio
SAP	Statistical analysis plan
SMQ	Standardized MedDRA query
WG	Working group
WHO	World Health Organization

FOREWORD

A medicinal product is expected to have a positive balance of benefits and risks (also referred to as favourable and unfavourable effects) at the time of authorization. However new potential harms may emerge (or existing risks may need to be better characterized) during the whole life cycle of a new product and older marketed drugs may be scrutinized for safety issues that may not have been recognized during development and their earlier years on the market.

Regulatory tools have been developed within pharmacovigilance over the last decades with the purpose of closely following up any safety issue that emerges following authorization and further evaluating potential or known risks of the product. Scientific tools that have been increasingly used for the evaluation of potential harms during the whole life cycle of a medicinal product are meta-analysis and systematic reviews. A safety meta-analysis is conducted to address whether the accumulated data indicate harm for a particular treatment or treatments. A usual purpose is to estimate an average effect for the studies at hand with the purpose of protecting future patients.

A broad range of challenging drug safety topics have been addressed within the CIOMS working groups, which have comprised expert senior scientists from regulatory authorities, the biopharmaceutical industry and academia. From the beginning the working groups (WGs) were focused on the processes for detection and management of potential problems during the development and use of drugs. The initial guidelines for international reporting of adverse events with a standardized "CIOMS I form" for standardized international reporting of individual cases of serious, unexpected adverse drug reactions in 1990 was followed by guidance on periodic safety update reports (known as "PSURs") and core data sheets.

Initially the WGs were concentrating on post-authorization processes but, as new WGs were formed, the scope was widened to include safety aspects of the whole life cycle of medicinal products. CIOMS WGs V, VI and VII covered areas such as pragmatic approaches in pharmacovigilance, management of safety information from clinical trials, and harmonization of the format and content for periodic safety update reports (PSURs) during clinical trials. This was followed by the CIOMS WG VIII report on signal detection, managing the life cycle of a signal including detection, prioritization and evaluation of a signal. The most recent publication, CIOMS WG IX's report, presents practical approaches to risk minimization for medicinal products.

In addressing the topic of meta-analysis and systematic reviews, this CIOMS WG X has met on a number of occasions in various locations hosted by the organizations or biopharmaceutical companies where some of the members of the WG hold positions (see Annex III). The members have worked to achieve consensus as far as possible and are alone responsible – in their capacity as experts – for the views expressed in this publication. These views do not necessarily represent the decisions, policies or views of their institutions or companies.

Although some of the content of this report describes highly technical statistical concepts and methods (in particular Chapter 4), the ambition of the working group has been to make it comprehensible to non-statisticians for its use in clinical epidemiology and regulatory science. To that end, Chapters 3 and 4, which contain the main technical statistical aspects of the appropriate design, analysis and reporting of a meta-analysis of safety data are followed by Chapter 5 with a thought process for evaluating the findings of a meta-analysis and how to communicate these.

All chapters and their content are further described in Chapter 1.

CHAPTER 1.

OVERVIEW AND INTRODUCTION

1.1 The subject

At the beginning of 2015, a general Google search [1] for "meta-analysis" yielded over 24 million hits, whereas a more specific PubMed search [2] for "meta-analysis" in the title of a scientific publication pointed to over 30 000 papers. This subject is almost an industry of its own! The field is much narrower, however, when the lens is limited to meta-analysis of adverse events (AEs) of "safety" or "harms" in the context of medicinal products intended for administration to humans. Nevertheless, this field is still very extensive. This report is about meta-analysis in this narrow area, but the present report should also provide conceptually helpful points to consider for a wider range of applications, such as vaccines, medical devices, veterinary medicines or even products that are combinations of medicinal products and medical devices. The goal of this report is to provide principles on appropriate application of meta-analysis in assessing safety of the above products to inform regulatory decision-making.

The term "meta-analysis" can have different meanings when used by different people. Other relevant terms are "systematic review", "overview" and "evidence synthesis". These terms are sometimes used interchangeably with "meta-analysis", although we, as do many scientists who currently work in the field, use the term "meta-analysis" to refer solely to the statistical aspects of combining evidence.

The CIOMS X Working Group has deliberately chosen to define "meta-analysis" in this context as:

> **The statistical combination of quantitative evidence from two or more studies to address common research questions, where the analytical methods appropriately take into account that the data are derived from multiple individual studies** (see Glossary).

There are a number of alternative definitions used by others, including previous CIOMS working groups, but this Working Group has agreed on the above as a simple, straightforward definition that covers the scope of the Working Group's interests.

This definition has been adopted for two key reasons:

▶ The concept of meta-analysis should not be constrained only to an activity that follows a systematic literature review. It requires careful selection criteria and inclusion of all relevant data. The principles in this report may be applied in situations where a single organization owns all of the data for a medicinal product.

▶ Meta-analysis should generally preserve within-study comparisons from the original studies; it is NOT "crude pooling" (which is adding up all the results for the treatment group, then adding all the results for the comparator group and comparing these summarized results). Many methods may be appropriate, such as generalized linear models, Bayesian methods and so on, as long as they do not ignore the fact that the data are derived from multiple studies.

A meta-analysis may be conducted at any time before or after a medicinal product is approved for marketing. For example, meta-analysis techniques should generally be utilized for the Integrated Summary of Safety that is included in the Common Technical Document at the time of a regulatory submission. Postmarketing of a medicinal product, there are regular mandated regulatory reviews, notably Periodic Safety Update

Reports (PSUR), also called Periodic Benefit-Risk Evaluation Reports (PBRERs), where meta-analysis may help, even if it is not required, to summarize data on outcomes following treatment when new studies are conducted during the reporting period [3], (see section 3.9 of this ICH guideline E2C (R2)).

For many clinically important questions, however, searching the literature and finding *all* of the relevant studies is a challenging, and possibly the most important, aspect of obtaining summary results from multiple studies. During premarketing drug development and in the registration process for an innovative product, this aspect may be of reduced relevance if all the studies, including individual participant data, are readily available. However, the selection criteria are of paramount importance; they impact on the strength and quality of evidence and, thus, the persuasiveness provided by a meta-analysis.

The principles for conducting a meta-analysis, as described in this report, are intended to be applied to a drug development programme in the regulatory setting at any phase of the product life cycle. Most of what we discuss focuses on a single (main) question, whereas drug development has many goals, including safety signal detection, which of necessity deals with many studies with multiple AEs and time points. It is important to use meta-analysis methods to assess the data, rather than crude pooling.

1.2 Overview and scope

Although there are many publications on meta-analysis, (e.g. [4-7]) the current practice and set of principles, such as those from the Cochrane Collaboration, are not sufficient on their own because they do not specifically address issues relative to the evidentiary criteria and persuasiveness of meta-analysis for regulatory decision-making, especially in drug safety. This report gives some broad explanation of the general methods for statistical or numerical synthesis of evidence but does not attempt to be a comprehensive textbook for this area.

Safety data may be combined from multiple clinical studies in different ways (if the strategy is sound). The following are examples that illustrate some of the situations where the principles in this report can be applied:

▶ A summary of observed events from a clinical development programme in an integrated analysis at time of product approval for marketing. Meta-analytical principles are generally recommended to be used (as opposed to crude pooling) for the comparison of treatment groups to assess AEs for the potential to be causally related to a drug.

▶ A prospective meta-analysis to assess a specific AE. An example is the evaluation of cardiovascular risk in the development of drugs for diabetes mellitus [8].

▶ A regulatory body or sponsor may initiate its own meta-analysis in response to safety signals raised by other investigators. This may be particularly useful for a regulatory body when it has access to data from several sponsors [9-12].

▶ Other investigators may initiate meta-analyses for various reasons (e.g. in response to a safety signal) [13-15].

▶ A summary of observational studies to evaluate safety endpoints. An example is a meta-analysis of observational data from 25 publications in 18 populations to assess the possible association of myocardial infarction and individual nonsteroidal anti-inflammatory drugs [16].

The following paragraphs in this section provide an introduction to each of the subsequent chapters in this report.

The primary goal of Chapter 2 is to provide background and context for the use of meta-analysis (and systematic reviews) in drug development and regulatory decision-making. The chapter concludes with a cautionary note that, while these evolving approaches can enhance understanding of medicine safety and contribute to overall benefit-risk assessments, care must be taken to evaluate strengths, data sources and methodological requirements. These all may ultimately have an impact on the regulatory decision-making process.

The goal of Chapter 3 is to describe how to design a meta-analysis of safety data that will yield meaningful and useful results. Emphasis is placed on the importance of prospectively planning meta-analysis protocols. The intent is to describe pragmatic principles for design that have situational flexibility, rather than to constrain stakeholders by providing strictly prescriptive rules. Topics addressed include defining the population of interest, study selection, outcome definition and validation, examining risk of bias in individual studies, and implications of using individual participant-level vs. summary-level data. The main emphasis of this report is on analysis of randomized trials but, in some instances, observational studies are able to provide the most important (or at least additional) evidence and Chapter 3 contains a section on specific issues in the meta-analysis of observational studies. Chapter 3 also contains a section that introduces the concept of network meta-analysis and discusses some of the important principles related to the topic of network meta-analysis. There is a great deal of stakeholder interest in this area but, in the view of the Working Group, this topic is not yet mature enough to provide comprehensive consensus guidance on how to perform and utilize such analyses.

The goal of Chapter 4 is to provide guidance on the analysis and reporting associated with meta-analyses of safety data. This chapter provides technical details on data analysis once design has been finalized and data have been collected. A checklist is included in section 4.10.2 that outlines the items that would be expected in a report of a meta-analysis. Extensive examination of these technical aspects is not in the scope of this chapter, as in-depth details are available elsewhere for those who may be interested. However, practical implications and importance of the analytical choices are described. This chapter is rather technical, although interpretive context is provided.

Chapter 5 is intended for the less technical reader and designed to describe a thought process for evaluating the findings of a meta-analysis. The recommended approach begins with first impressions, followed by a more thorough evaluation of the methodology, the fit with other evidence, and implications of the findings for potential regulatory actions. Key points in Chapter 5 include assessing the overall importance of the results before analysing details, engaging appropriate experts in the review, and providing context of the results in relation to other available information on the benefits and risks of the product. Importantly, the chapter describes the potential for bias in source data, methodology, result interpretation, selective reporting and publication bias that might have an impact on the value – i.e. persuasiveness – of the meta-analysis. Finally, the chapter addresses how perceived public health impact and strength of the conclusions influence the urgency and the medium for communicating results, including relevant updates, and the context of those results.

The goal of Chapter 6 is to focus on the resources needed to conduct a meaningful meta-analysis. Since a meta-analysis is complex and requires diverse technical expertise, the Working Group recommends that the appropriate experts be engaged from the very early planning stages. General references are provided to guide team decision-making, although flexibility is encouraged since the specific question(s) will dictate the expertise needed. In addition to scientific planning, a dedicated team repository is recommended to comply with Good Clinical Practice documentation guidelines. Since the appropriate search strategy and data sources are important criteria for success, this chapter provides introductory guidance along these lines. It is recommended that the scope of a proposed meta-analysis include consideration of public as well as proprietary data sources, as may be appropriate and available.

Appendices 1–4 provide examples of real meta-analyses (some of which are referred to within the body of the report) that illustrate issues that are discussed in this report.

A glossary, which is provided in Annex I, covers the specific terms and definitions that are of importance for, and used in, this report. However, neither the glossary itself nor the individual definitions can be regarded as comprehensive; they are included as an aid to the reader.

1.3   The readership

This report is aimed at a rather broad audience. Two key groups are regulatory authorities and those with drug safety responsibilities at biopharmaceutical companies. These stakeholders should find the report particularly useful. It is intended for those with experience in medical and scientific aspects of drug safety but who may have more limited formal statistical or epidemiologic training. The Working Group hopes that this report will enable these stakeholders to understand more of these latter aspects, as applied to meta-analysis. Another important stakeholder group is statisticians for whom the statistical methods are well-understood, but whose experience in assessing impactful AEs may be somewhat limited. Clearly, collaboration between these stakeholder groups will be important to concerned organizations and will benefit patient safety. At the very least, this report should enable the various stakeholder groups to communicate more clearly and to facilitate collaboration in producing high-quality meta-analyses, including considerations for understanding the strengths and limitations of combining data from several clinical studies.

It is also the hope of the Working Group that this report will be of interest to independent academics, contract research organizations, patient advocacy groups, practising health-care professionals, other scientists, and science writers when carrying out or critically evaluating studies in this field.

1.4   The future

This area continues to be of increasing importance, complexity continues to evolve, and the number of manuscripts published using meta-analysis is increasing dramatically. The move towards more "open" data and transparency in analysis will make increasing volumes of data available from expanding data sources available for analysis. This expansion of meta-analysis (not all of which will be well done or interpreted properly) will present challenges. The Working Group hopes that this report is timely in that sense and will underscore the need for high-quality work that ultimately translates to improved patient safety.

References Chapter 1

1. Google. Keyword "meta-analysis" searched 26 March 2015. www.google.com.
2. U.S. National Center for Biotechnology Information. PubMed advanced search builder; keyword "meta-analysis" searched 26 March 2015. http://www.ncbi.nlm.nih.gov/pubmed/advanced.
3. European Medicines Agency. ICH guideline E2C (R2) on periodic benefit-risk evaluation report (PBRER). 2013, EMA/CHMP/ICH/544553/1998, 1-45. http://www.ema.europa.eu/docs/en_GB/document_library/Regulatory_and_procedural_guideline/2012/12/WC500136402.pdf.
4. Borenstein M, Hedges LV, Higgins JP, Rothstein HR. Introduction to Meta-analysis. 2009, Chichester, UK: John Wiley & Sons.
5. Egger M, Smith GD, Altman D. Systematic reviews in health care: meta-analysis in context. 2nd ed. 2008, London, UK: John Wiley & Sons.
6. Higgins JP, Green S, eds. Cochrane Handbook for Systematic Reviews of Interventions Version 5.1.0 [updated March 2011]. 2011, The Cochrane Collaboration. http://handbook.cochrane.org/.
7. Khan K, Kunz R, Kleijnen J, Antes G. Systematic reviews to support evidence-based medicine. , 2011. 2nd ed. 2011, London, UK: Royal Society of Medicine.
8. U.S. Food and Drug Administration. Guidance for industry: Diabetes mellitus-evaluating cardiovascular risk in new antidiabetic therapies to treat Type 2 diabetes. 2008. http://www.fda.gov/downloads/Drugs/GuidanceComplianceRegulatoryInformation/Guidances/UCM071627.pdf.
9. Hammad TA, Laughren T, Racoosin J. Suicidality in pediatric patients treated with antidepressant drugs. Arch Gen Psychiatry, 2006, 63(3): 332-339.
10. Kim PW, Wu YT, Cooper C, Rochester G, Valappil T, Wang Y, Kornegay C, Nambiar S. Meta-analysis of a possible signal of increased mortality associated with cefepime use. Clin Infect Dis, 2010, 51(4): 381-389.
11. McMahon AW, Levenson MS, McEvoy BW, Mosholder AD, Murphy D. Age and risks of FDA-approved long-acting beta(2)-adrenergic receptor agonists. Pediatrics, 2011, 128(5): e1147-1154.
12. Colman E, Szarfman A, Wyeth J, Mosholder A, Jillapalli D, Levine J, Avigan M. An evaluation of a data mining signal for amyotrophic lateral sclerosis and statins detected in FDA's spontaneous adverse event reporting system. Pharmacoepidemiol Drug Saf, 2008, 17(11): 1068-1076.
13. Nissen SE, Wolski K. Effect of rosiglitazone on the risk of myocardial infarction and death from cardiovascular causes. N Engl J Med, 2007, 356(24): 2457-2471.
14. Nissen SE. Setting the RECORD straight. JAMA, 2010, 303(12): 1194-1195.
15. Singh S, Loke YK, Furberg CD. Inhaled anticholinergics and risk of major adverse cardiovascular events in patients with chronic obstructive pulmonary disease: a systematic review and meta-analysis. JAMA, 2008, 300(12): 1439-1450.
16. Varas-Lorenzo C, Riera-Guardia N, Calingaert B, Castellsague J, Salvo F, Nicotra F, Sturkenboom M, Perez-Gutthann S. Myocardial infarction and individual nonsteroidal anti-inflammatory drugs meta-analysis of observational studies. Pharmacoepidemiol Drug Saf, 2013, 22(6): 559-570.

CHAPTER 2.

BACKGROUND

The purpose of this chapter is to provide the regulatory and scientific context for the use of research synthesis at all stages in the life cycle of a drug. At any point in the drug development process, systematic reviews and meta-analysis can provide important information to guide the future path of the development programme and any actions that might be needed in the postmarketing setting. This chapter gives the rationale for why and when a meta-analysis should be considered. This is all in the context of regulatory decision-making, and the tasks, data collection, and analyses that need to be carried out to inform those decisions. Although this is the primary focus here, as noted in Chapter 1, we hope it will be useful outside the regulatory setting.

2.1   The context for this report

There is increasing demand by decision-makers in health care, the biopharmaceutical industry, and society at large to have access to the best available evidence on benefits and risks of medicinal products. The primary evidence is generally randomized controlled clinical trials (RCTs) used for the regulatory process. The best strategy will take an overview of all the evidence and where it is possible and sensible, combine the evidence and summarize the results. For efficacy, the outcomes generally use the same or very similar predefined events for each of the trials to be included. However, the (inevitably) unplanned nature of the data on safety makes the process more difficult.

Combining evidence on AEs, where these were not the focus of the original studies, is more challenging than combining evidence on pre-specified benefits. A variety of problems arise, notably in terms of multiple possible outcomes and multiple, possibly imprecise, definitions for particular outcomes other than all-cause mortality. This summarized evidence might help, in conjunction with other sources of evidence such as knowledge about other similar drugs or other studies, to decide whether particular AEs are likely to be associated with drug exposure. It is crucial to assess the importance of the harm in the context of benefit-risk of a particular product. (Note though that full scale assessment of the benefit-risk balance is beyond the scope of this report.)

Several guidelines for reporting systematic reviews and meta-analysis (as well as much other important information) are available at the EQUATOR site [17]. These include the PRISMA guidelines [18] for reporting meta-analysis as well as their extensions for individual patient data meta-analysis [19] and network meta-analysis [20]. While these guidelines focus on the reporting of meta-analysis rather than on their conduct, they have many aspects that are useful to consider when planning a meta-analysis.

Current regulatory guidance is rather sparse on aggregation and analysis of data to address a question that the original studies did not set out to answer. It is worth noting that most regulatory guidance and many Cochrane Collaboration reviews have usually given more attention to assessment of benefits, while issues around combining evidence on harms have not been as well-covered. The book by Khan et al. cited by reference [7] in section 1.2 above does have a chapter on the critical appraisal of harms using an example from a published review, but this approach in looking at harms specifically is uncommon. Our focus on AEs represents the main contribution of the current CIOMS report.

2.1.1 Current background of synthesis research

A history of "research synthesis" [21] quotes the physicist Rayleigh from 1885 as emphasizing the need not only for "the reception of new material" but "the digestion and assimilation of the old". The term "meta-analysis" was introduced in 1976 [22], though statistical methods for utilizing data from different studies had been used before. Although social scientists may have been ahead of medical researchers in 1976, the latter rapidly caught up with new statistical methods for combining data, especially from randomized clinical trials [23]. The Cochrane Collaboration (www.cochrane.org) has been pivotal both in drawing attention to the need for systematic reviews in health care, and also in actually carrying out the reviews and keeping them up-to-date. It has made a strong stand in terms of being independent from potentially biased stakeholders.

It is particularly relevant that the Cochrane Collaboration established a small, informal subgroup in 2001 to evaluate the harmful effects of interventions [24]. This subgroup, the Adverse Effects Methods Group (AEMG), was officially sanctioned in 2007 and has become a valuable resource for methodological guidance on best practice techniques for identification and systematic evaluation of adverse effects. The AEMG assumes that every intervention in health care has an associated potential for at least some harmful effects. The rate at which these harmful effects occur may be low and, if low, the statistical power to decide whether they are caused (or not) by the intervention (drug) at a genuinely higher (or convincingly not higher) rate than the comparator may be insufficient. This means that it will be difficult to decide on causation. Thus, for informed decision-making, systematic assessments of both benefits and harms of the intervention are needed. The AEMG provides scientific advice when methodological uncertainties arise, particularly related to harms of interventions. This group has also recognized that observational data may be relevant and that, for some questions, restriction of evidence only to that derived from RCTs is unnecessarily limiting.

The emphasis of meta-analysis is on reducing the random or sampling error, and may also shed some light on systematic variation in results. If the original trials have biases, recognized or not, then the meta-analysis may lead to directionally inappropriate conclusions because the apparent sampling variation has been reduced, perhaps dramatically so by meta-analysis, but the bias has been replicated in the studies. This is obviously a major problem for observational studies but even RCTs can be affected (e.g. by having inadequate follow-up time). There are also biases that can arise in the conduct of the meta-analysis itself, even if all the included studies are of high quality. An example of such bias, which has gained a lot of attention, is "publication bias". However, over-emphasis on the publication process as the source of bias may lead to neglect of other sources. (See section 3.8 for a discussion of potential sources of bias). It is of interest that, in a commentary in the Journal of the American Medical Association (JAMA), co-authored by one of the JAMA editors, the authors note, "Accordingly, JAMA considers meta-analysis to represent an observational design, such that outcomes, inferences, and interpretations should be described as associations rather than reported using causal terms" [25].

The history of the field includes those with strong opposition to performing meta-analysis on data not based on primary endpoints [21, 26, 27]. It has been recognized for some time that the reporting of harms in published clinical trial reports is inadequate, even though there are specific guidelines on this issue produced by the Consolidated Standards of Reporting Trials (CONSORT) Group [28]. The situation for trials used by regulators in evaluating drugs is that the quality should be as high as possible, but as soon as there is reliance on published data we need to be aware of relevant scientific caveats when looking at data evaluating harms [29].

Almost all of the above discussion relates to data from RCTs. There is little disagreement that, where the relevant question can be answered using data where allocation to treatment was random, such data should be preferred. Where uncertainty remains in spite of randomized data being available or where no data on an important question exist, data from observational studies may need to be utilized.

A good example of a situation where randomized data have been usefully supplemented by observational data is the question whether cyclooxygenase-2 (known as "COX-2") inhibitors increase the risk of cardiovascular harm. In reviewing data on COX-2 inhibitor-associated cardiovascular risk from 138 randomized trials, Kearney et al., estimated a summary relative risk (RR) of 1.42 (95% CI, 1.13-1.78) [30]. McGettigan et al. came to an essentially similar result of a summary RR of 1.31 (95% CI, 1.18-1.46) for rofecoxib based on a meta-analysis of observational studies [31]. More importantly, the observational data gave a summary RR of 2.19 (95% CI, 1.64-2.91) with rofecoxib doses above 25 mg per day, where the trial data were insufficient to make this calculation. The observational data also indicated that the risk may be increased early in treatment, whereas the trial data initially did not capture this time-to-hazard relationship. This finding was further confirmed by other observational studies [32].

A particularly strong example where meta-analysis of observational data has been very helpful is in the area of hormones. Randomized trials of combined oral contraceptives when comparing two active treatments would be possible, but it would not generally be ethical to compare them with placebo (because of the risk of unintended pregnancy in women exposed to placebo). Apart from ethical considerations, for very rare effects, the RCTs are generally inadequate and observational studies on, for example, the effect of combined oral contraceptives on risk of breast cancer, were very controversial. Partly at least, because of the controversy, Dr. Valerie Beral at Oxford University's Cancer Epidemiology Unit assembled a group of a large number of investigators [33] to integrate their individual data from the observational studies. She then showed a small absolute and relative risk associated with combined oral contraceptives [34].

Dr. Beral's group has also looked at hormone replacement therapy and risk of breast cancer, and they showed an advantage of having the individual data available. Beral showed that time since menopause may be more relevant than age. This analysis was possible, even though the original authors did not present such analyses, because the date of menopause was recorded in the data coming from the studies. It may be noted that the recent PRISMA statement on individual patient data (also sometimes called patient-level data, participant-level data, or individual-level data, and here abbreviated as IPD) addresses randomized trials and not observational data. It is clear that, although the statistical methods may be similar to those used for IPD meta-analysis using data from RCTs, the interpretation will have to be substantially more cautious [35-37].

2.2 The context of drug development and the regulatory process

During the development of a medicinal product, RCT data are collected, mainly designed to support claims of efficacy but also including safety-related information – such as AEs, laboratory data, patient reported outcomes, vital signs, electrocardiograms). All of these sources are important but we focus on information entered onto case report forms as AEs. Some AEs are actively collected because knowledge of pharmacology, class effects, or other information has led to the belief that they are important. The coding of AEs may also present some difficulties when they are not part of the outcomes defined carefully in the trial protocol. Further, many AEs are not (and cannot be) pre-specified, and are thus entered as free text, which is subsequently coded using a dictionary, such as Medical Dictionary for Regulatory Activities (MedDRA), to facilitate analysis.

The trial report will summarize those AEs and usually also will provide some statistical estimate of the magnitude of harms identified during the trial. Summaries of these data are produced for each study and for the overall development programme, but in many instances for regulatory purposes they are tabular and narrative rather than being formal statistical analyses. Interpretation based on simple tabular displays can be misleading, as discussed by Lièvre et al. [38] and Chuang-Stein & Beltangady [39] who show that displays utilizing crude pooling can be misleading.

For the purposes of assuring safety, there can be important limitations in RCT data. The type of patients excluded – such as those with comorbidities, severe disease, or hepatic or renal impairment – can have an impact on generalizability. If such patients are included, their numbers may be so small that it implies a meta-analysis may be helpful. Similarly, the duration of treatment and/or follow-up and restriction of dose may limit extrapolation but, if some data are available from individual studies, meta-analysis may help. Regulatory bodies, sponsors (in this context, the biopharmaceutical company sponsoring the trials in order to obtain a licence or marketing authorization) and investigators might use meta-analysis to summarize and combine data from multiple clinical studies to assess the safety of drugs, either before or after regulatory approval and marketing authorization.

It is worth noting that there is no absolute requirement for meta-analysis to be part of a regulatory submission. For example, the International Council for Harmonisation of Technical Requirements for Pharmaceuticals for Human Use (ICH) *Guideline E2F on the Development Safety Update Report* notes that data from a meta-analysis may "become available" and hence may contribute [40, section 3.10], but does not specifically suggest that meta-analyses should be conducted routinely. Similarly, ICH E9 remarks (although in the context of assessing efficacy) "meta-analysis may be informative", and notes also the need for a "prospectively written protocol" [41]. While there is no absolute requirement for meta-analysis to be part of drug development, the Working Group believes that meta-analysis should be part of ongoing safety surveillance and is generally advised to be part of regulatory submissions in situations where combining data is appropriate.

Meta-analyses of safety data can be performed before and after the marketing approval of a drug. A simplified schematic of the role of meta-analysis in assessment of clinical safety data for a medicinal product or class of products is shown in Figure 2.1. Meta-analyses done before marketing of a drug are undertaken to investigate AEs of special interest, for signal detection and to help inform on causality, to assess the necessity of risk management and risk minimization activities and to assess the benefit-risk balance of a drug (e.g. for progression decisions during development, for the dossier at time of submission, or for discussions between industry and regulators).

Meta-analyses done after marketing are usually undertaken to update safety information from clinical trials or to further investigate new safety findings. Postmarketing safety findings are often related to rare AEs which cannot be studied in a single clinical trial, or which are related to more common events when there may be a small excess in an already high background incidence (e.g. cardiac events). In these situations, larger numbers of exposed subjects are required to show a small treatment difference. New clinical trials are common after marketing - and meta-analyses can be undertaken with the results of these added to further delineate benefits and risks. Equally a meta-analysis can be used to generate hypotheses for further testing, in both efficacy and safety, as happened with the International Studies on Infarct Survival (known as "ISIS") [42-46] which investigated the effect of different treatments on mortality and major morbidity of patients with definite or suspected acute myocardial infarction.

Figure 2.1 Simplified schematic of the role of meta-analysis in assessment of clinical safety data for a medicinal product or class of products

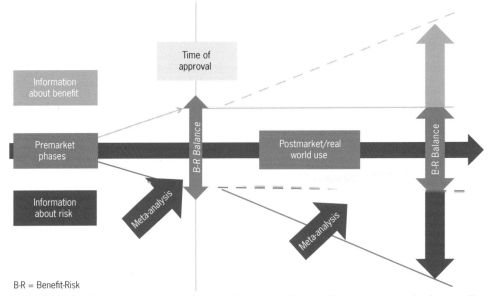

B-R = Benefit-Risk

Source: Adapted from Hammad et al. The future of population-based postmarket drug risk assessment: a regulator's perspective. Clin Pharmacol Ther, 2013 [47].

Many regulators are in the unique position of having all the relevant trials for an unlicensed product but, except at the US Food and Drug Administration (US FDA), there has not been a strong tradition of conducting meta-analyses. The potential for doing meta-analysis using individual participant data is obvious but not routine practice, and the resources required to assemble the data and carry out the analysis are very considerable - possibly requiring several (often two to five) person-years of effort. It is often the case that crude pooling (adding up all events in treatment and comparator groups, ignoring the fact that the results came from individual studies) of trial results is done in submissions by sponsors that is part of the New Drug Application dossier. Such crude pooling is generally discouraged as it can yield invalid results because of the potential for confounding by study [38, 39, 48 (Figure 1)]. Regulators do not routinely re-analyse these data, though it may be possible to do so.

Over the last decade many regulatory safety issues have been raised in meta-analyses that address possible drug-induced adverse effects. Meta-analyses have often added to the evidence and have informed decision-making on the safety of a medicinal product. However, such meta-analyses may also be a source of debate or even confusion when different analyses addressing the same question draw different conclusions (e.g. [10, 49]). This shows that there is a need for high standards in conducting meta-analysis.

Regulatory deliberations following a meta-analysis will sometimes result in a change to the regulator-approved prescribing information (e.g. U.S. Package Insert or EU Summary of Product Characteristics) but they can result in no change at all or, at the other extreme, in drug withdrawal from the market.

In addition to performing their own meta-analyses of safety data, regulatory authorities and biopharmaceutical sponsors are increasingly compelled to react to the results of meta-analyses that are published by researchers or civil society groups outside the regulatory field in the scientific literature or elsewhere. (Appendices 3 and 4 of this report are specific examples of cases where this occurred). Reacting in this context means assessing the quality and robustness of the meta-analysis, as well as the impact of the results on the benefit-risk balance of the product. This impact assessment may be framed by a regulatory decision made in the past or may inform, along with other sources of evidence, a future decision.

Meta-analysis of safety data can be expected to increase in frequency and have a higher profile in the media for various reasons, including greater transparency and more openness regarding data from both RCTs and postmarketing use of medicinal products.

Scientists in regulatory authorities, biopharmaceutical sponsors or other stakeholder organizations, including academic institutions, conduct meta-analyses. In principle, all these groups can conduct credible meta-analyses, but sometimes there is differential access to relevant trial data because of privacy or intellectual property concerns. Access to data can be a major driver for differing inclusion of various studies. If the studies to be included are different in alternative reviews, then it could lead to different results and, thus, to different conclusions.

It is clearly important to have access to results from **all** relevant studies, published or not, whatever the findings. There is controversy over whether investigators or trial sponsors, including industry, have made or should make available all such data, and over the next few years such availability of clinical trial data is likely to increase, though whether this will usually be based on individual records or summary data is not yet clear. The US Institute of Medicine has published a discussion setting out a possible framework on transparency and data-sharing [50, 51]. That committee published its report in January 2015 [52] coinciding with a number of industry sponsors who announced their intentions to release more unpublished data, at least for new trials, if not for trials conducted in the past. For example, several institutions announced a joint mechanism to access data through a website – Clinicalstudydatarequest.com [53] – and Yale University scientists are also collaborating with industry in sharing data through the Yale University Open Data Access (YODA) Project [54]. The industry trade associations in the USA and Europe, the Pharmaceutical Research and Manufacturers of America (PhRMA) and the European Federation of Pharmaceutical Industries and Associations (EFPIA), have made general commitments to transparency and data-sharing as described in the *Joint principles for responsible clinical trial data sharing* [55, 56].

The European Medicines Agency has taken a number of steps in this area, and published a press release entitled *European Medicines Agency policy on publication of clinical data for medicinal products for human use* in October 2014 [57, 58].

The appropriate process for sharing data at an individual level still needs to be worked out in detail. There are obvious concerns over privacy and the possibility of linkage to other sources of data leading to loss of confidentiality.

The overall consequences are that much more data will be available to those outside the biopharmaceutical industry in the future, and this report will offer some guidance to those who wish to analyse the data to evaluate drug safety. Individual sponsors typically already have data available in principle, though in practice it is not as easy as this sounds (for instance, with sponsor mergers the legacy computer systems cannot always easily extract the relevant data or with some investigator-sponsored trials the data may not be available).

Both the CIOMS Working Group VI [59] and the Safety Planning, Evaluation and Reporting Team (SPERT) [60] suggested that sponsors implement a well-defined, coordinated, programme-wide approach to identify safety signals early in the drug development process. SPERT further recommended that this include the creation of a prospectively defined "Program Safety Analysis Plan (PSAP)". SPERT gave advice for planning for meta-analysis, understanding that many safety questions are best answered by meta-analysis of RCT data. The CIOMS Working Group VI also gave suggestions for the use of meta-analysis in the context of drug development in Chapter 6 of their report.

2.3 Why do we need to synthesize evidence?

In nearly all biological and medical research a single study rarely provides a definitive answer to the relevant questions. Even if the answer to the intended question of a single study has been answered unequivocally, the data collected might be repurposed to answer other questions. The latter use may have some philosophical objections, but there is a need to make optimum use of available data, since data are generally expensive in time, resources and commitment of investigators and of research participants. Thus, it might be argued that there is an ethical imperative to make optimum use of those data by exploring all their appropriate uses.

It is vital that stringent attention be paid to evaluating the safety of medicinal products both before and after a product is authorized for marketing. The assessment of evidence for safety will usually need to encompass the totality of data on the possible harms of the medicine, in the context of expected benefits, so that some synthesis of the evidence will need to be done. It is also critical to identify important gaps in information about adverse effects that may not have been looked for and were not detected in early trials, or that may occur in subgroups of patients who were not included in the development programme. An example of a knowledge gap that is increasingly receiving attention is the lack of insight into patient perspectives and preferences about acceptable trade-offs regarding a specific safety issue, given an expected level of benefit [61]. This gap might stem from lack of adequate engagement of patients in determining what endpoints are important to measure. Such missing information will result in uncertainty on safety in the context of possible uses of the medicinal product in daily medical practice. Full coverage of the issues arising in practice is out of the scope of this report

2.4 Important considerations for research synthesis

RCTs have the potential to support strong causal inference – i.e. in the safety context, to support that the drug causes an event as opposed to being associated with an event. (The latter can happen readily in observational studies.) Because the treatment allocation is random in RCTs, known and unknown factors by which subjects differ are balanced out. Bias reduction has been addressed in many ways in randomized trials, but even randomized trials are not immune from bias. For example, missing data (e.g. from dropouts) can introduce bias to the interpretation of answers to important questions. The choice of the studies to include, the extraction of the relevant data (and deciding what is, and what is not "relevant") are all issues where bias can be introduced.

Rather more on bias will be found in the next chapter of this report (section 3.8). Much work has been done by the Cochrane Collaboration on the risk of bias in randomized trials. Chapter 8 of the Cochrane Handbook [6] is completely devoted to this issue.

In addition there is a tool that looks at the different important domains in which bias can arise [62] and this tool has been used a great deal in Cochrane reviews. A generic bias assessment tool may not be sufficient in any given situation, as there may be clinical or study design issues relevant to a particular therapeutic question. There remains controversy over whether or not the source of funding should be included in any checklist of risk of bias [63, 64].

Traditional methods of meta-analysis attempt to combine results in order to obtain a single summary of effect size. It is important to consider to what extent the results of studies are consistent, because different patient characteristics can result in differing responses to therapy. In this situation, a single summary number may be quite inadequate. See section 4.8 for information regarding heterogeneity and how to investigate it.

In principle, RCTs have clearly-specified protocols that define all aspects of the design, execution, data collection, analysis and reporting of a trial. The primary outcome (in some trials more than one outcome is primary) is pre-specified, so that the potential for post-hoc rationalization and choice of data to report is limited. In practice, it does not always work like this for trials that are published, though those trials used for regulatory submissions tend to have strict adherence to the protocol. There is evidence that other trials, even those of supposedly high quality where the protocols were submitted to, and accepted by, peer-reviewed scientific journals, may not adhere to the protocol when it comes to the final published report [65]. Similar problems of discrepancy between protocol and final publication can occur with meta-analyses [66]. There may be good reasons to change a protocol for any form of research, but all such changes should be documented. The fact that such discrepancies exist shows that there is potential for bias, both in the original trials and also in meta-analyses of those trials. Naive interpretation must therefore be avoided.

For published randomized trials, the extraction of the numbers with and without the event in each treatment arm of the trial should in theory be simple. Binary data are the types of data that are most often used in relation to issues of safety. These numbers may not be given in a publication, but the data should be available to both regulators and sponsors. In some publications, recurrent events are reported as if they were independent. However, care must be taken when extracting data to ensure that, for the purposes of most meta-analyses, it is the count of patients with (at least one) event that is given and not the number of events. Cochrane review groups have large teams and spend many months doing a single review. This also shows that just checking that a meta-analysis has been done correctly is not simple. Recalculating the summary statistics from a given table is fairly easy, but being sure that the numbers in the table are correct requires major effort. With observational studies it may be much more difficult to extract (and check) the relevant data.

2.5 Conclusions

Systematic review and meta-analysis of safety data have become well-known features in the life cycle of many medicinal products. Indeed, these approaches are evolving into very sophisticated methods that enhance understanding of the safety profile of medicines and can make important contributions to overall benefit-risk assessments. However, meta-analyses may have different strengths, data sources, methodological requirements and impact on the regulatory decision-making process. Thus, care must be taken in all aspects of the design, data selection, methodological approach and interpretive criteria for the results of a meta-analysis to have maximal impact on protection of patient safety.

References Chapter 2

6. Higgins JPT, Green S, eds. Cochrane Handbook for Systematic Reviews of Interventions Version 5.1.0 [updated March 2011]. 2011, The Cochrane Collaboration. http://handbook.cochrane.org/.

7. Khan K, Kunz R, Kleijnen J, Antes G. Systematic reviews to support evidence-based medicine. , 2011. 2nd ed. 2011, London, UK: Royal Society of Medicine.

10. Kim PW, Wu YT, Cooper C, Rochester G, Valappil T, Wang Y, Kornegay C, Nambiar S. Meta-analysis of a possible signal of increased mortality associated with cefepime use. Clin Infect Dis, 2010, 51(4): 381-389.

17. EQUATOR Enhancing the QUAlity and Transparency Of health Research. A comprehensive searchable database of reporting guidelines. www.equator-network.org.

18. Moher D, Liberati A, Tetzlaff J, Altman DG, PRISMA Group. Preferred reporting items for systematic reviews and meta-analyses: the PRISMA statement. J Clin Epidemiol, 2009, 62(10): 1006-1012.

19. Stewart LA, Clarke M, Rovers M, Riley RD, Simmonds M, Stewart G, Tierney JF, Group P-ID. Preferred Reporting Items for Systematic Review and Meta-Analyses of individual participant data: the PRISMA-IPD Statement. JAMA, 2015, 313(16): 1657-1665.

20. Hutton B, Salanti G, Caldwell DM, Chaimani A, Schmid CH, Cameron C, Ioannidis JP, Straus S, Thorlund K, Jansen JP, Mulrow C, Catala-Lopez F, Gotzsche PC, Dickersin K, Boutron I, Altman DG, Moher D. The PRISMA extension statement for reporting of systematic reviews incorporating network meta-analyses of health care interventions: checklist and explanations. Ann Intern Med, 2015, 162(11): 777-784.

21. Chalmers I, Hedges LV, Cooper H. A brief history of research synthesis. Eval Health Prof, 2002, 25(1): 12-37.

22. Glass GV. Primary, Secondary, and Meta-Analysis of Research. Educ Res, 1976, 5, 3-8. http://www.jstor.org/stable/1174772.

23. Baber NS, Lewis JA. Beta-blockers in the treatment of myocardial infarction. BMJ, 1980, 281(6232): 59.

24. Cochrane Collaboration. Cochrane Adverse Effects Methods Group. 2007, The Group aims to develop the methods for producing high quality systematic reviews and to advise the Cochrane Collaboration on how the validity and precision of systematic reviews can be improved. http://aemg.cochrane.org/.

25. Berlin JA, Golub RM. Meta-analysis as evidence: building a better pyramid. JAMA, 2014, 312(6): 603-606.

26. Eysenck HJ. Meta-analysis and its problems. BMJ, 1994, 309(6957): 789-792.

27. Shapiro S. Meta-analysis/Shmeta-analysis. Am J Epidemiol, 1994, 140(9): 771-778.

28. Ioannidis JP, Evans SJ, Gotzsche PC, O'Neill RT, Altman DG, Schulz K, Moher D, Group C. Better reporting of harms in randomized trials: an extension of the CONSORT statement. Ann Intern Med, 2004, 141(10): 781-788.

29. Hodkinson A, Kirkham JJ, Tudur-Smith C, Gamble C. Reporting of harms data in RCTs: a systematic review of empirical assessments against the CONSORT harms extension. BMJ open, 2013, 3(9): e003436.

30. Kearney PM, Baigent C, Godwin J, Halls H, Emberson JR, Patrono C. Do selective cyclo-oxygenase-2 inhibitors and traditional non-steroidal anti-inflammatory drugs increase the risk of atherothrombosis? Meta-analysis of randomised trials. BMJ, 2006, 332(7553): 1302-1308.

31. McGettigan P, Henry D. Cardiovascular risk and inhibition of cyclooxygenase: a systematic review of the observational studies of selective and nonselective inhibitors of cyclooxygenase 2. JAMA, 2006, 296(13): 1633-1644.

32. Hammad TA, Graham DJ, Staffa JA, Kornegay CJ, Dal Pan GJ. Onset of acute myocardial infarction after use of non-steroidal anti-inflammatory drugs. Pharmacoepidemiol Drug Saf, 2008, 17(4): 315-321.

33. Oxford University. Cancer Epidemiology Unit. 2015. http://www.ceu.ox.ac.uk/team/valerie-beral.

34. Collaborative Group on Hormonal Factors in Breast Cancer. Breast cancer and hormonal contraceptives: collaborative reanalysis of individual data on 53 297 women with breast cancer and 100 239 women without breast cancer from 54 epidemiological studies. Lancet, 1996, 347(9017): 1713-1727.

35. Beral V, Banks E, Reeves G, Wallis M. Hormone replacement therapy and high incidence of breast cancer between mammographic screens. Lancet, 1997, 349(9058): 1103-1104.

36. Collaborative Group on Hormonal Factors in Breast C. Familial breast cancer: collaborative reanalysis of individual data from 52 epidemiological studies including 58,209 women with breast cancer and 101,986 women without the disease. Lancet, 2001, 358(9291): 1389-1399.

37. International Collaboration of Epidemiological Studies of Cervical C, Appleby P, Beral V, Berrington de Gonzalez A, Colin D, Franceschi S, Goodhill A, Green J, Peto J, Plummer M, Sweetland S. Cervical cancer and hormonal contraceptives: collaborative reanalysis of individual data for 16,573 women with cervical cancer and 35,509 women without cervical cancer from 24 epidemiological studies. Lancet, 2007, 370(9599): 1609-1621.

38. Lièvre M, Cucherat M, Leizorovicz A. Pooling, meta-analysis, and the evaluation of drug safety. Curr Control Trials Cardiovasc Med, 2002, 3(1): 6.

39. Chuang-Stein C, Beltangady M. Reporting cumulative proportion of subjects with an adverse event based on data from multiple studies. Pharmaceut Statist, 2011, 10(1): 3-7.

40. European Medicines Agency. ICH guideline E2F on development safety update report. 2010. http://www.ema.europa.eu/docs/en_GB/document_library/Scientific_guideline/2010/09/WC500097061.pdf.

41. ICH International Conference on Harmonisation. ICH E9 Statistical principles for clinical trials ICH Harmonised Tripartite Guideline. 1995. http://www.ich.org/products/guidelines/efficacy/efficacy-single/article/statistical-principles-for-clinical-trials.html.

42. ISIS-4 (International Study of Infarct Survival). ISIS-4: a randomised factorial trial assessing early oral captopril, oral mononitrate, and intravenous magnesium sulphate in 58,050 patients with suspected acute myocardial infarction. ISIS-4 (Fourth International Study of Infarct Survival) Collaborative Group. Lancet, 1995, 345(8951): 669-685.

43. ISIS-3 (International Study of Infarct Survival). ISIS-3: a randomised comparison of streptokinase vs tissue plasminogen activator vs anistreplase and of aspirin plus heparin vs aspirin alone among 41,299 cases of suspected acute myocardial infarction. ISIS-3 (Third International Study of Infarct Survival) Collaborative Group. Lancet, 1992, 339(8796): 753-770.

44. ISIS-2 (International Study of Infarct Survival). Randomised trial of intravenous streptokinase, oral aspirin, both, or neither among 17,187 cases of suspected acute myocardial infarction: ISIS-2. ISIS-2 Second International Study of Infarct Survival) Collaborative Group. Lancet, 1988, 2(8607): 349-360.

45. ISIS-1 (International Study of Infarct Survival). Randomised trial of intravenous atenolol among 16 027 cases of suspected acute myocardial infarction: ISIS-1. First International Study of Infarct Survival Collaborative Group. Lancet, 1986, 2(8498): 57-66.

46. Fourth International Study of Infarct Survival: protocol for a large simple study of the effects of oral mononitrate, of oral captopril, and of intravenous magnesium. ISIS-4 collaborative group. Am J Cardiol, 1991, 68(14): 87D-100D.

47. Hammad TA, Neyarapally GA, Iyasu S, Staffa JA, Dal Pan G. The future of population-based postmarket drug risk assessment: a regulator's perspective. Clin Pharmacol Ther, 2013, 94(3): 349-358.

48. Hammad TA, Pinheiro SP, Neyarapally GA. Secondary use of randomized controlled trials to evaluate drug safety: a review of methodological considerations. Clin Trials, 2011, 8(5): 559-570.

49. Kalil AC. Is cefepime safe for clinical use? A Bayesian viewpoint. J Antimicrob Chemother, 2011, 66(6): 1207-1209.

50. Institute of Medicine. Discussion Framework for Clinical Trial Data Sharing: Guiding Principles, Elements, and Activities. 2014, Washington, DC: The National Academies Press.

51. Olson S, Downey AS, Institute of Medicine (U.S.). Forum on Drug Discovery Development and Translation, Institute of Medicine (U.S.). Forum on Neuroscience and Nervous System Disorders, National Cancer Policy Forum (U.S.), Institute of Medicine (U.S.). Roundtable on Translating Genomic-Based Research for Health, Institute of Medicine (U.S.). Board on Health Sciences Policy, Institute of Medicine (U.S.). Board on Health Care Services. Sharing clinical research data : workshop summary. 2013, Washington, D.C.: The National Academies Press.

52. Institute of Medicine. Sharing Clinical Trial Data: Maximizing Benefits, Minimizing Risk. 2015. http://iom.nationalacademies.org/Reports/2015/Sharing-Clinical-Trial-Data.aspx.

53. Wellcome Trust. ClinicalStudyDataRequest.com. 2014, The Wellcome Trust has taken responsibility for managing the review of research proposals and the operation of the Independent review panel (IRP). The Trust will also administer the IRP secretariat and appoint new panel members. www.wellcome.ac.uk. https://www.clinicalstudydatarequest.com/.

54. Yale School of Medicine. Yale University Open Data Access (YODA) Project. 2015. http://yoda.yale.edu/welcome-yoda-project.

55. Pharmaceutical Research and Manufacturers of America (PhRMA). PhRMA Principles For Responsible Clinical Trial Data Sharing. 2013. http://www.phrma.org/phrmapedia/responsible-clinical-trial-data-sharing.

56. European Federation of Pharmaceutical Industries and Associations (EFPIA). Joint Principles for Responsible Clinical Trial Data Sharing to Benefit Patients. 2013. http://transparency.efpia.eu/clinical-trials.

57. European Medicines Agency. European Medicines Agency policy on publication of clinical data for medicinal products for human use. 2014. http://www.ema.europa.eu/docs/en_GB/document_library/Other/2014/10/WC500174796.pdf.

58. European Medicines Agency. Questions and answers on the European Medicines Agency policy on publication of clinical data for medicinal products for human use. 2015. http://www.ema.europa.eu/docs/en_GB/document_library/Report/2014/10/WC500174378.pdf.

59. CIOMS Working Group VI. Management of Safety Information from Clinical Trials. 2005, Geneva: Council for International Organizations of Medical Sciences.

60. Crowe BJ, Xia HA, Berlin JA, Watson DJ, Shi H, Lin SL, Kuebler J, Schriver RC, Santanello NC, Rochester G, Porter JB, Oster M, Mehrotra DV, Li Z, King EC, Harpur ES, Hall DB. Recommendations for safety planning, data collection, evaluation and reporting during drug, biologic and vaccine development: a report of the safety planning, evaluation, and reporting team. Clin Trials, 2009, 6(5): 430-440.

61. Hammad TA, Neyarapally GA. Legislative Policy [BJC1] and Science Considerations in the Era of Patient-Centeredness, Big Data, and Value. in Benefit-Risk Assessment Methods in Medicinal Product Development: Bridging Qualitative and Quantitative Assessments, 1st. 2016, CRC Press Taylor and Francis Group: Boca Raton, FL.

62. Higgins JP, Altman DG, Gotzsche PC, Juni P, Moher D, Oxman AD, Savovic J, Schulz KF, Weeks L, Sterne JA, Cochrane Bias Methods G, Cochrane Statistical Methods G. The Cochrane Collaboration's tool for assessing risk of bias in randomised trials. BMJ, 2011, 343: d5928.

63. Bero L. Editorial: Why the Cochrane risk of bias tool should include funding source as a standard item. 2013. http://www.cochranelibrary.com/editorial/10.1002/14651858.ED000075.

64. Sterne JA. Editorial: Why the Cochrane risk of bias tool should **not** include funding source as a standard item. 2013. http://www.cochranelibrary.com/editorial/10.1002/14651858.ED000076.

65. Al-Marzouki S, Roberts I, Evans S, Marshall T. Selective reporting in clinical trials: analysis of trial protocols accepted by The Lancet. Lancet, 2008, 372(9634): 201.

66. Dwan K, Gamble C, Williamson PR, Kirkham JJ, Reporting Bias G. Systematic review of the empirical evidence of study publication bias and outcome reporting bias - an updated review. PLoS One, 2013, 8(7): e66844.

CHAPTER 3.

PLANNING

This chapter begins with a brief description of two different types of meta-analyses: retrospective meta-analysis and prospective meta-analysis. It is followed by a list of the elements that define a complete protocol in a preparation for a meta-analysis. The ensuing sections focus on specific aspects of design that are particularly relevant to assessing safety in the regulatory context, including:

— 3.1 Preparing for the meta-analysis

— 3.2 Definition of population of interest

— 3.3 Definition of outcomes

— 3.4 Trials of different durations

— 3.5 Study selection and data extraction

— 3.6 Study size and small study effects

— 3.7 Multi-arm trials

— 3.8 Risk of bias of the meta-analysis, individual study and overall

— 3.9 Access to individual participant data, summary-level data, or both

— 3.10 Specific issues in meta-analysis of observational studies

— 3.11 Network meta-analysis

3.1   Preparing for the meta-analysis

Summary of main points:

▶ There are particular issues unique to meta-analysis for drug safety evaluation in the regulatory setting, such as prospective planning of a programme-level meta-analysis, access to individual participant data for meta-analysis of RCTs, and the distinction between exploratory and confirmatory meta-analysis.

▶ There is a spectrum of different types of meta-analyses from retrospective meta-analysis to prospective meta-analysis. Prospective meta-analysis can help overcome some of the recognized problems of retrospective meta-analyses and offers many advantages.

▶ Regardless of the type of meta-analysis, a well-thought-out, prospectively planned protocol is always needed in order to guide the conduct of meta-analysis. A detailed statistical analysis plan (SAP) should be constructed along with the protocol.

▶ Some main elements in the design of meta-analysis should be included in a meta-analysis protocol.

▶ Publication of a protocol for the systematic review prior to knowledge of the available studies reduces the impact of review authors' biases, and promotes transparency, which is important. An international registry of systematic review protocols has recently been established at the Centre for Reviews and Dissemination at the University of York, UK, in collaboration with the U.K. National Health System's National Institute for Health Research [67]. When the meta-analysis is being conducted with a subsequent publication planned, the protocol should be registered.

▶ While the intention should be that the meta-analysis will adhere to the published protocol, changes in a protocol are sometimes necessary. It is important that changes in the protocol not be made on the basis of how they affect the findings of the research study. All changes to the protocol for the meta-analysis should be fully documented and a rationale for each change should be provided.

Although there is a large collection of literature on meta-analysis, the current practice and set of principles, such as those from the Cochrane Collaboration, are not sufficient on their own because they do not specifically address issues relative to the evidentiary criteria and persuasiveness of meta-analysis for regulatory decision-making, especially in drug safety. This chapter describes the main elements in the design of meta-analysis that should be part of the meta-analysis protocol, which is considered the first step in the process before the analysis is undertaken. The intent is not to repeat the existing, well-established meta-analysis principles in great detail; rather, the particular issues unique to meta-analysis for drug safety evaluation in the regulatory setting will be highlighted and emphasized – such as prospective planning of a programme-level meta-analysis, access to individual participant data for meta-analysis of RCTs, and the distinction between exploratory and confirmatory meta-analysis.

Meta-analyses are often performed retrospectively on studies that have not been planned with the goal of meta-analysis in mind. (One of the goals of this report is to move meta-analysis further in the direction of being prospective.) In addition, many meta-analyses are based solely on summary statistics that have been extracted from published papers. In this document, we shall refer to meta-analyses (that are planned and performed on studies for which the results are already known) as retrospective meta-analysis. A prospective meta-analysis is a meta-analysis of studies, generally RCTs, identified, evaluated and determined to be eligible for the meta-analysis before the results of any of those trials become known [6].

Prospective meta-analysis can help overcome some of the recognized problems of retrospective meta-analyses by enabling hypotheses to be specified *a priori*; prospective application of selection criteria for trials and prospectively defined analysis plans, before the results of the trials are known. This avoids potentially biased, data-dependent emphasis on particular subgroups or endpoints. The prospective meta-analysis approach offers other advantages. A key advantage is the potential for prospective and rigorous collection of the outcome data. Additionally, many prospective meta-analyses will analyse IPD. The use of patient-level, as opposed to summary-level, data offers many advantages, such as facilitating the exploration of heterogeneity at the patient level and permitting analyses of time-to-events (see more details in section 3.9). A prospective meta-analysis can be planned to have adequate statistical power to study questions that could not be addressed in individual studies (e.g. uncommon clinical outcomes, safety endpoints and planned subgroup analyses). Having plans in place to publish those analyses, regardless of the findings, is a main step in avoiding publication bias. Standardization of data collection across studies is also facilitated with prospective meta-analysis [60].

A special case of a prospective meta-analysis is when the component trials themselves are planned to be used in the meta-analysis so they can be designed to provide an unbiased treatment effect estimate for the outcome of interest. An example of this is described in the US FDA draft guidance for industry, *Diabetes mellitus: Developing drugs and therapeutic biologics for treatment and prevention (2008)* [8].

In truth, there is a spectrum of meta-analyses from retrospective to prospective. In situations where the meta-analysis includes some studies where the results are known in advance and others where they are not known in advance, it would be advisable to include results both separately and overall. Related to this spectrum, the meta-analysis may have IPD for some studies and only summary-level data for others. Statistical methods have been developed to combine these [68, 69].

As a study of studies, it is logical that meta-analysis should be guided by study design principles similar to those of other research activities. Regardless of the type of meta-analysis, a protocol is always needed in order to guide the conduct of meta-analysis. A well-thought-out protocol also can help clarify expectations, enhance transparency, rigor and validity, and promote a consistent approach for meta-analysis. At a minimum, even when all the data exist, one still needs a protocol that will define the main parts of the meta-analysis (e.g. the kind of studies, the inclusion and exclusion criteria, the statistical analysis plan, etc.).

In retrospective meta-analysis in particular, prior knowledge of the results of a potentially eligible study may, for example, influence the definition of a systematic review question, the subsequent criteria for study eligibility, and the choice of intervention comparisons to analyse, or the outcomes to be reported in the review. Because of this opportunity for the introduction of bias, it is important that the investigators establish and document all methodological decisions in advance. Additionally, publication of a protocol for a review prior to knowledge of the available studies reduces the impact of the review authors' biases, promotes transparency of methods and processes, reduces the potential for duplication, and allows peer review of the planned methods [70]. An international registry of systematic review protocols, called PROSPERO, was established in 2011 at the Centre for Reviews and Dissemination at the University of York, United Kingdom [67].

Detailed descriptions of what belongs in a meta-analysis protocol are available in multiple existing publications (e.g. the Cochrane Handbook) [6]. For the sake of completeness, we offer a high-level presentation here, and then go on to focus on specific aspects of design that are particularly relevant to assessing safety in the regulatory context.

A meta-analysis protocol should include, but is not limited to, the following elements:

- **Background:** This section describes the regulatory context and reasons for undertaking a meta-analysis. It provides an overview of the study treatment, including mechanism of action, indications and doses. The section should provide a brief overview of what is known about the state of evidence for the safety issue to be evaluated and should clearly indicate whether the results of certain trials are known.

- **Objectives:** This section states the objectives that will define the scope and nature of the meta-analysis. A statement of the review's objectives should begin with a precise statement of the primary objective, followed by one or more secondary objectives. The research question should specify the types of population (participants), types of interventions (and comparisons), and the types of outcomes that are of interest. The acronym PICO (Participants, Interventions, Comparisons, Outcomes) helps to serve as a reminder of these. Some authors have expanded PICO to PICOS or PICOTS, with "T" standing for timing and "S" representing either "study design" or "setting".

- **Eligibility criteria:** Eligibility criteria are a combination of aspects of the research question plus specification of the types of studies that have addressed these questions. The aspects include study population, treatment (or, more broadly, intervention), comparisons, outcomes and study type.

- **Definition, harmonization and adjudication of outcomes of interest (called outcomes in the following):** This section specifically defines the outcomes. It provides details of criteria for combinability of subjects, treatments (doses), outcomes and lengths of follow-up; describes procedures for assessment of outcomes (e.g. blinded to treatment assignment); distinguishes between studies designed to assess the outcome and studies in which the outcome was assessed after study completion. Composite outcomes should be handled with caution with a thoughtful justification of the use of such an outcome and of the individual components. In relation to the definition of outcomes, either the protocol or a separate document should specify the charter and adjudication procedure for clinical expert committees in order to minimize bias in case ascertainment.

- **Sources of data and study selection:** This section defines the procedures for identifying and finding all the relevant studies (both published and unpublished) to be included in the meta-analysis and the procedures for abstracting the relevant data from the selected studies (including the number of planned abstractors).

- **Assessment of the opportunity for bias in the individual studies:** This section describes the methodology for assessment of the study designs and assessing potential biases.

▶ **Statistical analysis plan:** A detailed SAP should be constructed along with the protocol. (Note: A detailed discussion of analysis methods is presented in Chapter 4). The SAP should specify:

— Primary analysis population (e.g. intention-to-treat, as-treated or per protocol). Arguments are sometimes made in favour of using a "per protocol" population for a safety question or an "as-treated" analysis. All these populations can be biased for assessment of safety [59, 71-76].

— What to do in case the preferred population is not available. In addition to the primary analyses, one should identify populations for important sensitivity analyses. One sensitivity analysis (if it is not the primary analysis) should correspond to minimal selection decisions – in other words, using as much data as possible from the original trials and imposing as few opinions of the meta-analysts as possible. Only then does it become obvious what effect these opinions have.

— Operational definitions of variables and pertinent coding dictionaries.

— Plans to examine balance in follow-up times and pertinent confounders between comparator groups, within each trial.

— Handling of missing data at the subject or summary level.

— Choice of summary effect measures (e.g. risk difference, odds ratio, or risk ratio).

— Details of statistical methodologies.

— Plans for assessment of any important assumptions of the statistical model.

— Any subgroup analyses to be performed and plans to examine balance in risk factor distributions in subgroups between the comparator groups within each trial.

— (Optional) Power to rule out a specified degree of increased risk. This could be accomplished by displaying power plots that cover a plausible range of a values showing how sample sizes relate to detectable alternatives of risk estimates [77].

— Handling of sparse data or zero event trials.

— If Bayesian approaches are used, providing details on assumptions, choice of priors and sensitivity analysis relating to prior specification, implementation and result reporting.

— Plans for sensitivity analyses.

▶ **Clinical and statistical heterogeneity:** This section describes the approach to assessing statistical and clinical heterogeneity, discusses the properties of the statistical methodology selected (fixed-effect vs. random-effects models), and determines the study level and subject level covariates to be explored (e.g. via meta-regression).

▶ **Plans to present and report results:** Here, for example, the plan may include displaying the summary data from each study, and overall, graphically (forest plots). Both point estimates and interval estimates should be included. Planned publications should also be detailed.

Meta-analysis protocols should, in general, be registered. While the intention should be that the meta-analysis or systematic review will adhere to the published protocol, changes in a protocol are sometimes necessary. This is similarly the case for a protocol for a randomized trial, which must sometimes be changed to adapt to unanticipated circumstances such as problems with participant recruitment, data collection or unexpected event rates. While every effort should be made to adhere to the predetermined protocol, this is not always possible or appropriate. It is important, however, that changes in the protocol not be made on the basis of how they affect the findings of the research study. Post hoc decisions made when the impact on the results of the research is known, such as excluding selected studies from the meta-analysis or systematic review, make the study findings highly susceptible to bias and should be avoided. All changes to the protocol for the meta-analysis, as with amendments to clinical trials protocols, should be fully documented and a rationale for each change should be provided in a form that enables complete transparency, including in any published reports.

Having defined the protocol elements at a high level, the rest of this chapter focuses on a subset of the elements that the authors believe are particularly challenging in the context of safety meta-analyses in the regulatory setting.

3.2   Definition of population of interest

Summary of main point:

▸ The population of interest should be defined before specifying the study search strategy, in order to avoid the introduction of bias.

Before specifying the study search strategy, the participant population of interest needs to be defined. This step is crucial in order to avoid the introduction of bias and to increase the likelihood that decisions taken on the basis of the study findings are applied to the appropriate population. The protocol should describe the set of subjects to be included in the primary and main secondary analyses, including specification of demographic and important baseline attributes that are potentially relevant to the outcome of interest. For example, if one wishes the analysis to focus on high-risk populations, the protocol should specify how "high-risk" is defined.

The criteria for which populations (and therefore which studies) should be included in a review have been well described in the Cochrane Handbook [6]. In general, the criteria should be sufficiently broad to encompass the likely diversity of patients treated in clinical practice, but sufficiently narrow to ensure that a meaningful answer can be obtained when studies are considered in aggregate. An important step is to define the broad population and settings of interest. This involves deciding whether a special population group is of interest, which might be based on factors such as age and sex, race, or the presence of a particular aspect of the disease being treated (e.g. "severe" disease or presence of a particular symptom, such as angina or shortness of breath). Interest may focus on particular settings, such as a community, hospitals, nursing homes, chronic care institutions or outpatient settings. Box 3.1 below shows Box 5.2a from the Cochrane Handbook [6] which outlines some factors to consider when developing criteria for the "types of participants".

The types of participants of interest usually determine directly the participant-related eligibility criteria for including studies. However, pre-specification of rules for dealing with studies that only partially address the population of interest can be challenging. For example, if interest focuses on children who are 16 years of age or younger, pre-specifying an upper limit of 16 years of age would not determine a strategy for dealing with studies with participants aged from 12 to 18 years. In this case a phrase such as "the majority of participants are under 16" might suffice. Although there is a risk of review authors' biases affecting post hoc inclusion decisions, this may be outweighed by a common sense strategy in which eligibility decisions keep faith with the objectives of the review rather than with arbitrary rules. Difficult decisions should be documented in the review, and sensitivity analyses can assess the impact of these decisions on the review's findings. (Of course, the best solution would be to have access to IPD, allowing the meta-analyst to select the *specific* participants of interest from a given trial.) [6]

Any restrictions with respect to specific population characteristics or settings should be based on a sound rationale, and that rationale should be specified in the protocol. When it is uncertain whether there are important differences in effects among various subgroups of people, it may be best to include all of the relevant subgroups and then test for important and plausible differences in effect in the analysis (see section 4.8 on Subgroup Analysis). This should be planned *a priori* and stated as a secondary objective [6].

Box 3.1 Factors to consider when developing criteria for types of participants.

> ▶ How is the disease/condition defined?
>
> ▶ What are the most important characteristics that describe these people (participants)?
>
> ▶ Are there any relevant demographic factors (e.g. age, sex, ethnicity)?
>
> ▶ What is the setting (e.g. hospital, community, etc.)?
>
> ▶ Who should make the diagnosis?
>
> ▶ Are there other types of people who should be excluded from the review (because they are likely to react to the intervention in a different way)?
>
> ▶ How will studies involving only a subset of relevant participants be handled?

Source: Box 5.2a of the Cochrane Handbook [6]. Used with permission of the publishers.

The factors discussed above will affect the generalizability of the meta-analysis results to particular populations using the medicinal product (to determine who should avoid the product).

3.3   Definition of outcomes

Summary of main points:

▶ Clear specifications of the adequate measurement of important safety outcomes are required.

▶ A composite outcome should be used when it makes biological sense and the protocol should include a thoughtful justification of the choice of such an outcome.

▶ RCTs, predominantly designed to study drug efficacy, are rarely designed and powered to evaluate drug safety and hence often lack a pre-specified systematic method of AE collection (e.g. some clinical concepts could be captured and coded differently). The first step in the evaluation of a post hoc meta-analysis is to examine whether there was adjudication and validation as well as ascertainment efforts for the safety outcome of interest.

In this section we discuss particular considerations in the definition of outcomes for prospective and retrospective meta-analyses. We begin with prospective meta-analyses since retrospective meta-analyses should, as far as possible, adhere to the same standards as prospective meta-analyses [6].

3.3.1   Defining outcomes for prospective meta-analyses

Prospective meta-analyses can be initiated during a drug development programme or during postmarketing with a consortium that collaborates on several studies. Prospective meta-analyses allow issues germane to outcome definition to be taken into consideration during the protocol writing and study conduct phases. These issues pertain mainly to outcome choice and validation and to how data are collected and adjudicated if needed.

Historically, broad searches for terms (or broad definitions of outcomes) were used to ensure that all relevant terms were included in the definition of the safety outcome. Use of broad composite outcomes, however, can also lead to an underestimation of the true relative risk and to potential masking of a safety signal/problem [60, 78] when the misclassification is "non-differential" – i.e. equally likely to occur in each treatment arm. Suppose that one has a particular interest in an event that may be expressed clinically as a spectrum of disease. A narrow classification may include only those events at the more serious end of the clinical spectrum, but a broad classification may include the entire clinical spectrum. The broader classification may include events that are less likely to be related to the true (but possibly unknown) mechanism of action or that, by their nature, are simply more likely to be misclassified in clinical trials. Under these circumstances, the observed relative risk will be closer to unity for the broader classification than for the narrower classification. For an interesting example see Chapter 9 of the book *Statistical methods for monitoring clinical trials* [79].

Outcome choice and validation

In general, clear specifications of the adequate measurement of important safety outcomes are required (e.g. for myocardial infarction, it might be important to ensure that cardiac enzymes are measured). When available, standard medical definitions of outcomes should be used. If there is no well-established definition in the medical literature, it may be important to obtain agreement from relevant regulatory bodies and other stakeholders on the use of a nonstandard definition. A validation effort also should be undertaken to evaluate the clinical relevance of the selected definition. It is worth noting that operational challenges might hinder the ability to evaluate the performance of a particular diagnostic algorithm due to lack of pertinent information that was not collected during the trial.

Use of surrogate outcomes

Surrogate outcomes (e.g. elevated liver enzymes as a surrogate for potential liver injury) are discouraged when sufficient information on the clinical outcomes is available. They add another layer of variability as they are one step removed from the intended outcomes. Furthermore, their validation is challenging (if even possible).

Use of composite outcomes

In general, composite outcomes should be used with caution. If used, the composite outcome should make biological sense and the protocol should include a thoughtful justification of the choice of such an outcome. The plan should also include analysis of individual components if composite outcomes are used. It is particularly important to identify situations where the overall result is driven by one of the components or where some of the components can go in a different direction from others. In effect, if the risk of one component increases and another decreases, the overall evaluation of the composite outcome might show no association. An additional consideration is how the definition of the composite outcome has an impact on the sensitivity and specificity of results of analysis of the particular AE of interest, which has an impact on the ability to detect and evaluate the relationships between the drugs and AEs.

Data collection and adjudication

Some safety outcomes may require the development of an event-specific case report form (CRF). The case definition could include information from the event-specific CRF and other information (e.g. MedDRA terms, laboratory values [80]). In some cases, protocols may require the collection of additional and more-detailed data for subjects with a suspected AE to facilitate the case identification and safety assessment. For example, a specific definition of a venous thrombotic event (usually including deep vein thrombosis and pulmonary embolism) may require some form of diagnostic confirmation (e.g. venography). Routine AE reports of a venous thrombotic event, provided by an investigator, may not always include the requisite confirmatory evidence. Early identification of venous thrombotic events as AEs of special interest would lead to generation of a specific CRF designed to collect the results of the confirmatory test, avoiding the need to retrieve medical records, which may not be complete, especially if information needs to be retrieved retrospectively.

In some situations, adjudication may be considered necessary. For example, an excess of hepatic events noted in Phase II could prompt denoting these as adjudicated events for Phase III. In such cases, an expert or group of experts (an adjudication committee) provides a medical classification and standardized evaluation of AEs. Ideally, adjudication is done prospectively; pre-specification and keeping the committee blinded to treatment status greatly strengthens the quality and credibility of the adjudication. Retrospective adjudication is generally more challenging than prospective adjudication, as the detailed clinical information required for the adjudication committee is easier to capture completely when defined prospectively. When adjudication is done across a development programme, it is probably wise to use the same adjudication committee across all trials within the programme in order to enhance consistency.

3.3.2 Defining outcomes for retrospective meta-analyses

The majority of meta-analysis in the literature is conducted post hoc. The same principles discussed with prospective meta-analyses apply; however, by virtue of relying on completed trials, some modifications to the principles are necessary. An effort should be made to acknowledge the operational challenges and to evaluate potential impact on the interpretation of findings. It is still important to specify clear definitions of the outcomes of interest in the meta-analysis protocol. However, operational challenges might hinder the ability to evaluate the performance of a particular diagnostic algorithm due to lack of pertinent information that was not collected during the trial.

Ideally, when basing a meta-analysis on published literature, the meta-analysis protocol should include a plan to contact individual study authors to understand the circumstances surrounding data on outcomes. For retrospective meta-analyses that might have access to individual participant data, it may be helpful to utilize these data to further understand and better define the outcomes collected in these trials.

The first step in a post hoc IPD meta-analysis is to plan for adjudication and validation as well as ascertainment effort. Hammad et al. [48] wrote:

> RCTs, predominantly designed to study drug efficacy, are rarely designed and powered to evaluate drug safety and hence often lack a pre-specified systematic uniform mechanism of AE collection. Due to the unexpected nature of many AEs, establishment of an a priori AE definition and use of tools specifically designed to ascertain AEs is often challenging, highlighting the importance of outcome ascertainment and validation efforts. For example, in a meta-analysis of antidepressant RCTs conducted to evaluate the association between antidepressant drugs and suicidality [81] among adolescents [9], investigators developed an evaluation scheme [82] to search and adjudicate suicidality events. This led to the discovery and/or reclassification of a significant number of AEs in the trials used to conduct the meta-analysis. This underscores the fact that differences in the methods of case ascertainment as well as those related to the completeness of clinical narratives may also result in substantial and unmeasurable differences across trials.

(Note that suicidality is now called "suicidal ideation and behaviour").

For a cross-sponsor meta-analysis, all aspects of the protocol should be discussed between regulators, sponsors, and those actually implementing the analysis (either the regulator or a neutral third party). Governance (decision-making authority) needs to be agreed in advance, whether it is the regulator or a steering committee made up of academic investigators. The sponsors will generally have a major role in preparing the data in a common format and may be included in discussions of the analysis plan, although not necessarily with decision-making power. As noted above, to the extent that the same adjudication committee can be used for all trials, consistency should be improved. Planning adjudication of outcomes in completed studies, where access to IPD is available, should take into consideration the level of documentation likely to be available to support the classification of events. Ideally, one would want enough information in the medical records to make the diagnosis based on clearly-defined clinical criteria. At a minimum, the accuracy of the medical codes should be checked so as to decide, for example, that the coded event is not intended to rule out a diagnosis. The charter for the adjudication committee should clearly specify the "rules" to be used in making adjudication decisions, and particularly how decisions will be made if definitive confirmatory clinical data are not available (e.g. how much reliance will be put on the clinical judgement of the treating physicians as reflected in the medical records). We note that decisions on adjudication can have a major impact on results of statistical analyses. If events are included that may not be true events, an adverse treatment effect could be masked. If the adjudication criteria are too narrow, specificity will be high, but the lack of sensitivity may mean that events are missed, which can also lead to bias and lack of statistical power.

3.4   Trials of different durations

Summary of main points:

▶ As a general principle, length of treatment or observation time should not be an exclusion criterion in a meta-analysis.

▶ Clinical studies of varying lengths of treatment and/or observation time might be informative in addressing the time course of an increase in risk.

▶ In a summary-level meta-analysis, the overall measure of risk and the association between the measure of risk and study duration should be assessed and the results should be given in the meta-analysis to help elucidate the pattern of risk over time.

▶ In a patient-level meta-analysis, survival analysis methods can be used to estimate the overall hazard ratio and the dependence of the hazard ratio on time.

As a general principle, length of study (treatment duration and/or observation time) should not be an exclusion criterion in a meta-analysis, particularly in the case where there is no *a priori* knowledge of the time course of excess risk. However, in some cases, *a priori* knowledge or clinical considerations can lead to a specific clinical safety question that imposes restrictions on study length. For example, meta-analysis might exclude studies shorter than a pre-specified minimum treatment duration, when there is clear expectation based on biological considerations that adverse effects should not be evident with such short duration of treatment. Similarly, the clinical question might concern the mortality risk of say, immediate-release calcium channel blockers in the 30 days after an acute myocardial infarction (MI). Mortality past this acute setting of 30 days would tend to mask any acute risk. However, safety meta-analyses in the regulatory setting are often conducted to address the general question of a possible increase in the risk of an AE on a particular treatment. From that perspective, clinical studies of varying lengths of treatment and/or observation time might be useful in addressing the question.

Once the set of studies to be included in the meta-analysis is determined by the clinical question, the analysis plan to produce summary measure of risk (e.g. incidence rate ratio, odds ratio, risk ratio, risk or rate difference) and 95% confidence interval (CI) should be developed, with plans to calculate estimates over the set of studies. When the meta-analysis is conducted on summary-level data, the association between the measure of risk and study duration should be assessed. This association could be analysed either by analysing studies of similar duration in separate subgroups or by using study duration as a covariate in a meta-regression model. It should be noted that the perception of how risk is changing with duration of exposure can be related to the analytical approach. For example, when the hazard ratio is constant over time, the relative risk for longer-duration studies will be less than that of shorter-duration studies, while the odds ratio for longer-duration studies will be greater than that of shorter-duration studies. Thus, a relative risk or odds ratio that depends on study duration does not necessarily imply that the hazard ratio depends on duration.

However, when incidence rates are small, which is almost always the setting that leads to a regulatory safety meta-analysis, incidence rate ratios, relative risks or odds ratios that decrease significantly with study duration are consistent with a decreasing hazard ratio over time, while the reverse pattern is consistent with an increasing hazard ratio over time. Even if the hazard ratio (or other measure of increased risk) varies with study duration, the summary measure of increased risk still yields a valid overall test of association of the event with treatment. However, reporting only the overall summary odds ratio is not sufficient when it varies with study duration. A short-term increase in risk during early exposure could be masked by mixing studies with extended follow-up with studies with short-term follow-up and reporting only the summary odds ratio. Similarly, an increase in risk that appears only after extended exposure and extended follow-up could be masked by mixing in short-term studies with the longer-term studies. The finding of the association with study duration should be given in the meta-analysis report along with the analytical results (e.g. summary odds ratios by study duration strata). The association with study duration would be a secondary finding, but would help elucidate the pattern of risk over time.

Meta-analyses are also conducted on individual participant data, where the time of the event is known for patients with an event and total observation time is known for patients without an event. These data allow flexibility in choosing observation times for analysis. For example, because the full data are available, it is possible to set a common observation time, "T", for all studies – i.e. patients with observation time greater than T are censored at time T. Limiting the analysis to time ≤ T can be useful for answering certain kinds of clinical questions and may avoid issues associated with long-term observation time, such as increased levels of dropout.

As noted previously, a big part of the decision regarding the way in which studies of different duration are included in a meta-analysis depends on the clinical question (long-term or short-term risk), mechanism of action (risk is during treatment or extends after treatment is stopped), and dropout pattern (potential for biased censoring in longer-term trials). Whether or not a common time is selected for analysis, if survival analysis is planned there are two important issues to consider. One is whether or not it is reasonable for the hazard ratio to be constant over time. The other is the potential for informative censoring. Informative censoring occurs when patients who are censored at a given time are at a higher (or lower) subsequent risk of an event than those patients in the same risk set who are not censored. Informative censoring will bias the estimate of the hazard ratio. For instance, in oncology studies, where patients are often treated with the study drug until progression of disease, the potential for informative censoring is high as patients on the study drug are at a higher risk for a study drug-related AE than those not on the study drug. Thus, a standard survival analysis is problematic unless a common observation time is chosen (at least within each study) where most patients are still on study drug. Another subtle issue that can often arise in clinical development is that when studies have extended observation time, which may either be on or off drug, sometimes it is hard to determine in the published manuscript if the event summaries pertain only to on-therapy events or to events in all the follow-up.

One other note of caution is warranted. In some situations, duration of treatment (or follow-up) may be confounded with other aspects of study design or study populations. For example, a shorter-term treatment might be studied in patients with more severe disease, while longer-term studies were conducted in patients with less severe disease. In such situations, care is needed in interpretation, since differences between results of short-term and long-term studies may be due to the duration of treatment per se or to the underlying severity of disease.

3.5   Study selection and data extraction

Summary of main points:

▶ Main factors influencing the selection of RCTs to be included in a meta-analysis of safety data are population(s) of interest and study design features, such as comparator, dose, duration, and methods of eliciting AEs (active vs. passive).

▶ It is generally most appropriate to combine data from studies that are similar (though not necessarily identical) with respect to these features.

3.5.1 Study selection

The selection of studies to be included in a meta-analysis lays the foundation for the evidence base that will be synthesized and therefore may affect the overall results. Study selection could affect not only the nature of the findings but also the generalizability of those findings to specific populations. Unlike efficacy outcomes, AE outcomes in clinical trials are seldom well-structured or defined *a priori*. This makes selection of studies for a meta-analysis of AEs more challenging [83].

Selection of studies includes considerations based on the population(s) of interest (as noted in section 3.2), as well as on study design features. Several features will be important to consider – such as dose, duration, methods of eliciting AEs (active vs. passive) and population – as it is generally most appropriate to combine data from studies that are similar (though not necessarily identical) with respect to these features. Such similarity may not be required for a meta-analysis when the (adverse) effects of treatment do not depend on the trial characteristics being considered. Whether that dependence exists or not is partly a theoretical question based on what we know about the biology of the disease and the mechanism of action of the drug(s), but can also be empirically-based, as described in the sections on heterogeneity (section 4.8). A thorough review of each individual trial protocol should be undertaken before deciding which subsets of studies are eligible to be combined. It is worth noting that the mere fact that several studies have similar initial protocols might not guarantee that the studies, as implemented, are similar. The actual execution of the protocols may differ from one study to another [48]. It is prudent to examine the data eventually collected to verify the conformance with pertinent inclusion and exclusion criteria, for instance [9].

Caution should be exercised with study protocols that direct investigators to document information only on AEs suspected to be drug-related . The International Conference on Harmonisation (ICH-E3) guidelines *Structure and content of clinical study reports* direct investigators to report all AEs that patients experience, notwithstanding the investigators' judgement on whether the AEs are drug-related [84, 85]. Specifically, we recommend analysing all AEs that are reported, and not limiting analyses to events considered to be drug-related by the original investigators. If there is a compelling reason to present such an analysis, the reason for including studies that are limited to AEs considered by the investigators to be drug-related should be explicitly stated.

Furthermore, the rigour of various studies might be driven by the point in the product's life cycle at which the study was conducted. Conceivably, there might be unmeasured differences between studies conducted in Phase III vs. other phases, those conducted by a competitor drug sponsor, and so on. Depending on how many studies are available, it might be prudent to present the findings separately according to various design attributes, including the known purpose of the study, to examine the potential impact of these differences on the overall meta-analysis findings; in effect separating, whenever feasible, data that suggested the safety problem from data that are used to evaluate that problem.

Studies of a given drug may also include different doses. One must decide whether to include all doses, possibly modelling dose-response relationships, to focus on the dose(s) to be marketed, or to examine higher-than-marketed doses to understand the risks of overdose (or lower-than-recommended doses to assess dose-response effects). Whatever the choice, the decision should be documented and justified in the protocol.

Indication for treatment is another topic that deserves special consideration. One needs to specify whether all indications for a particular drug will be included in a single analysis, or whether indications will be analysed separately. The decision depends on whether there is reason to believe that the treatment will affect the risk of AEs equally across indications, or there is prior reason to believe that different populations (indications) will respond differently to treatment with respect to AEs [9].

A decision should be made early on whether the investigation will focus only on one drug within a class, the whole class, or several classes of drugs. The rationale for the decisions should be made clear *a priori* and not be data-driven. For example, a decision might be based on similar mechanisms of action or chemistry or similar indications, and so on.

When a meta-analysis is to include data available in publications, the meta-analysis should always be preceded by a systematic review of all available research. This consideration would not apply to special situations in which, for instance, a sponsor is conducting a meta-analysis on a product that is not available on the market, or is conducting an analysis of its own trial data for which individual-level data are required for the analysis.

Expert guidance publications on conducting systematic reviews and meta-analyses of efficacy data include advice on the selection of studies, such as the Cochrane Handbook [6]. Several publications have discussed various aspects of systematic reviews and meta-analyses of AEs and safety data to some extent [6, 48, 60, 83, 86, 87]. For example, the Cochrane Adverse Effects Methods Group [87] and the Safety Planning, Evaluation and Reporting Team (SPERT), provide specific guidance related to meta-analyses of AEs and safety data [60]. Other pertinent guidance documents include the ICH M4E published by the International

Conference on Harmonisation [88], the US FDA's *Guidance on premarketing risk assessment* [89], and the report from CIOMS Working Group VI [59].

Rather than reiterating the complete study selection process, which has been fully developed and illustrated in the Cochrane Handbook [6], the following paragraphs focus on a few specific situations reviewers may encounter in study selection specific to the context and issues of AE evaluation.

Situation 1: One approach to creating a set of studies for meta-analysis would be to include only studies that are very similar in design, dose, patient population, etc., so as to help reduce variability in the resulting estimates of treatment effects. Alternatively, heterogeneity of designs and populations could be explicitly examined as a goal of the meta-analysis by being more broadly inclusive of studies and analysing relationships between study characteristics and study findings (see section 4.8 on heterogeneity). In such situations, careful attention needs to be paid to potential confounding of study-level factors with each other. For example, high-dose studies may have been conducted only in patients with more severe disease, making it impossible to know whether differences in results stem from the higher dose or the more severe disease.

Situation 2: A related common situation that should be considered in study selection is the selection of trials where the treatment groups represent different dose levels of the same compound. Meta-analyses in which all dose groups are combined will usually not be very informative. It would be sensible to create a primary group that excludes the higher- or lower-than-approved dose arms from the main grouping of placebo-controlled studies to characterize AEs from labelled indications (and labelled doses). Then, high-dose studies (arms) can be included in a secondary group in an effort to assess what could happen in the high dose range (i.e. possible overdose). In general, it is recommended to exclude dose arms that are lower than the market-authorized dose, as these may dilute the effects seen at the higher dose levels. However, events that may occur in the lower-dose studies should not be ignored and can be explored when the dose-response relationship is of interest.

The decision on whether to separate, or not, different dose arms depends also on the kind of AEs under study as these might be subject to different dose-effect relationships. For example, hypersensitivity reactions or anaphylactoid reactions can also occur with very low doses. For these events, exclusion of low-dose arms would not be appropriate.

Situation 3: One of the problems with a meta-analysis for safety data is that events are missing for many reasons. Sometimes the manuscript will restrict reporting to more frequently occurring events (e.g. "we only reported events with >=2% incidence in the treated group"), and sometimes we really do not know what the rules were for exclusion. The rules for exclusion may be different from study to study, so it is not just a matter of including/excluding the double zero studies. There can be a much bigger problem with missing data. Section 4.2 provides detailed information on how to deal with studies with zero events, and limitations associated with each approach.

Situation 4: Duration of treatment and/or duration of follow-up may also vary across trials. Depending on the type of AEs, one might expect acute effects (e.g. for anaphylactic and anaphylactoid reactions) that might occur early during follow-up, perhaps even on the first dose. In contrast, some events (e.g. malignancy) might occur only after a long duration of treatment or follow-up, perhaps because there is a long latency period between exposure and expression of the event.

Situation 5: It is often the case that more than two treatment groups have been included in some or all of the studies to be combined in meta-analysis. How to address the pair-wise comparisons when a multi-arm trial is included in meta-analysis will be discussed in section 3.7.

Situation 6: Only a proportion of research projects are published in sources that are easily identifiable, particularly in the case of investigational drugs. As such, performing meta-analyses of the published literature will be limited by the data that have been published. If the dissemination of research findings is influenced by the nature and direction of results, publication biases may arise. Biases also exist in the language of publication so that searches based on databases indexing primarily English and a few other languages may produce misleading results [90]. Section 3.8 discusses more about how to address the publication bias.

Situation 7: Results from flexible-dosing trials might summarize exposure data using the modal dose. Consider the scenario where a patient who tolerated a particular dose is assigned to a higher dosage. If an AE occurs, the patient is likely to be returned to the previous lower dose. Because the lower dose is likely to be the modal dose for this patient, the AE will be incorrectly linked to the lower dose, masking any dose-effect response. Incidentally, it is also conceivable that patients who require higher doses of medication may be generally sicker and more likely to develop AEs related to the underlying illness or its complications. Therefore, in this scenario, dose-effect evaluation may mistakenly attribute the higher rate of AEs to the higher dose [48].

3.5.2 Data extraction

In some situations, the only results available from randomized trials will be in published papers, or other publicly-available sources that do not provide access to individual participant-level data. For example, an academic investigator might be interested in developing a better understanding of a particular safety concern. (See Appendix 4 Case study on rosiglitazone.) In such situations, care needs to be taken to ensure accurate data abstraction from the publication. Data extraction errors are common and have been documented in numerous studies, some of which are described in the Institute of Medicine's book on systematic reviews [91]. For example, Jones and colleagues (2005) documented data extraction errors in 20 reviews (48%), some of which changed the summary results (but did not affect the overall conclusions) [92].

The process of data extraction is not well studied, particularly with respect to ways to improve accuracy and efficiency. One study found that experience with systematic reviews did not appear to affect error rates. Error rates were high (28.3–31.2%) regardless of experience [93]. A commonly-recommended strategy for reducing data extraction errors is to have two individuals independently extract data. In a pilot study, Buscemi and colleagues compared the rate of errors using a single reviewer with the rate using two independent reviewers to perform data extraction. For the single reviewer, a second reviewer checked the extracted data for accuracy and completeness, with any discrepancies resolved in subsequent conference [94] . With two reviewers, each individual independently extracted the data and then similarly resolved discrepancies through discussion. The single reviewer data extraction was faster but resulted in 21.7% more errors. Experts recommend that two data extractors should be used whenever possible (e.g. IOM). The Cochrane Collaboration also supports this view [6, Chapter 7]. The Centre for Reviews and Dissemination (CRD) at the University of York, United Kingdom, allows for the option that one individual could extract the data if a second individual independently checks for accuracy and completeness [95].

Please note that this section focuses only on conducting meta-analysis of randomized clinical trials, which provide good data on well-recognized, easily detectable adverse effects. However, the systematic evaluation of new, rare or long-term adverse effects, which are unlikely to be observed in clinical trials, may require the inclusion of other study designs: cohort, case-control, cross-sectional, and even case reports or case series. Section 3.10 provides a more detailed discussion on the issues related to meta-analysis of observational studies.

3.6 Study size and small study effects

Summary of main points:

▶ A general principle of meta-analysis is to include all studies, regardless of size, that address the research question of interest.

▶ Two important points to consider in the meta-analysis of studies of disparate sizes are the weights given to the individual study estimates in the meta-analysis and the consistency of the estimate(s) from the large trial(s) with the estimates from the small trials.

▶ Sensitivity analyses based on the choice of study weights and post hoc analyses of subgroups of studies based on the results of the heterogeneity analyses should be conducted to obtain a full understanding of the data.

Still under the broad topic of study inclusion, we next turn to situations in which there may be a mix of some very small and some very large studies. This is important, since large studies (as we will see in Chapter 4) can dominate a meta-analysis result in terms of the information they provide. Thus, a regulatory decision might, in effect, be driven by a single study, making it crucial to understand the freedom from bias in that single study. The overriding principle of meta-analysis is the inclusion of all studies that address the research question of interest. The rationale is that the summation or synthesis of study-specific effects over all studies might yield a better estimate of the treatment effect compared with any of the individual studies alone. This rationale should hold whether or not the studies are estimating a common effect, although there may be situations in which estimating a single effect obscures important information (see section 4.8 on heterogeneity).

As a result of this principle, the size of a study would be expected, at least in theory, to be of secondary importance to the inclusion criteria. That is, there may be many reasons why a study does not adequately address the research question of interest, but size alone might not be one of them. The advantage of meta-analysis, in fact, is exactly to overcome the sample size problems of individual studies. However, size may be related to the ability of an individual study to capture the event of interest. In the context of this chapter, size refers to the amount of information and not necessarily sample size. For example, a study in a relatively small sample of subjects with a high background incidence rate of the AE of interest may yield more events than a larger study in subjects with a low background incidence rate. If the parameter of interest is relative risk, then the study with smaller sample size in the situation with a high background rate has more information. The designation of study size based on the number of events should be made on the basis of the overall number of events, blinded to the within-treatment numbers.

Two important points to consider in the meta-analysis of studies of disparate sizes are:

▶ The method by which the information from many smaller trials and a large trial(s) are synthesized into an overall treatment estimate. This is a question of what weight to give to the individual study estimates in the meta-analysis.

▶ The consistency of the estimate(s) from the large trial(s) with the estimates from the small trials. This is a specific question (contrast) under the umbrella of heterogeneity of results.

In planning the meta-analysis with respect to sample sizes of the component studies, one has also to consider the planned analysis, as the analytical choice can influence the results. The most common weights, used when study is viewed as a fixed effect (see section 4.3 "Choice of statistical model"), are the inverses of the variances of the study-specific estimate of interest. (Note, however, as pointed out in section 4.2, inverse-variance weights are generally a poor choice when the event is rare.) The inverse-variance weights will yield an overall estimate with minimum variance, but would be dominated by the estimate(s) in the larger trial(s). For example, in meta-analysis of cardiovascular effects in 14 clinical trials, one study contributed 57% of the weight in estimating the overall odds ratio [96].

Other weights can be chosen *a priori*. For example, in order to mitigate the large trial dominance, equal weights (as in a typical arithmetic average) could be selected. However, equal weights will increase the variance of the overall estimate. Whether it is appropriate or not to give equal weights to the small and large trials is also open to discussion and should be evaluated on a case-by-case basis [97]. The rationale for the choice should be clearly specified in the meta-analysis protocol.

Other approaches are possible to dealing with situations in which there are many small trials and a small number (possibly one) of large trials. For example, one might obtain an overall estimate from the many small trials by the inverse variance method and combine this estimate with the estimate(s) from the large trial(s) by the equal weight method. One could then more directly compare the small-trial estimate with the large-trial estimate(s).

In random-effects models, the inverse variance weights include an estimate of the variability among studies of the study-specific estimates. This leads to more uniform weights for the individual studies than does the fixed-effect model. However it is recommended that the fixed-effect vs. random-effects model be determined by the research question (see section 4.3.1) and not as a method for addressing the many small trials/ large outcome trial issue. When the results of the two approaches vary substantially, more effort should be made to understand the source of the difference between the two approaches.

In summary, all studies that address the research question of interest, regardless of study size, should be included in the meta-analysis. In the case where there are many small trials and relatively few large trials, the primary study weights to determine the overall treatment estimate and the tests of heterogeneity should be specified in the methods section of the meta-analysis protocol. Sensitivity analyses based on the choice of study weights and post hoc analyses of subgroups of studies based on the results of the heterogeneity analyses should be conducted to obtain a full understanding of the data.

There are two additional points to raise in the context of a discussion of trial size. The first point concerns the relative quality of small and large trials. While study size may be suggestive of higher quality it is not necessarily the case that bigger equals better. For example, as stated by Berlin & Kim regarding the anti-tuberculosis vaccine Bacillus Calmette–Guérin (known as the "BCG vaccine") [98]: "… for BCG vaccine, a huge trial using passive follow-up, and therefore missing (by the authors' own admission) at least 50% of all cases of tuberculosis, failed to show the protective effect found in a number of other studies with more complete follow-up" [99, 100]. Berlin & Kim also point out that large trials are subject to heterogeneity of results. They state: "Another paper [101] points out that one can also find discrepancies between large trials of the same therapy." They found that, in approximately 27% of pairs of large studies identified from the Cochrane Library, the two studies had findings that were statistically significantly different from each other.

This is identical to the proportion of discrepant comparisons in a highly visible paper by LeLorier [102] in which comparisons between meta-analyses and subsequent large trials were made. A related issue has to do with a post hoc meta-analysis effort that might encounter many small studies that could have been exploratory in nature. This may, in effect, overwhelm the point estimate of the meta-analysis in a direction that does not reflect the true nature of the relationship between the drug and safety issue of interest; a potential for a sort of "volume bias" might be encountered [47].

The second point comes from a regulatory perspective, where size may also refer to the size of a development programme. The research question of interest may be concerned with the safety of a class of drugs. Assigning weights to studies within a development programme and weights across development programmes to obtain an estimate of the class effect should take into account the size of the development programme. More detailed discussions can be found in some examples (e.g. selective serotonin reuptake inhibitors (SSRIs) and suicidality [9], and antiepileptic drugs and suicidality) [103]. The appropriateness of estimating a class effect is a question in some situations owing to the possible heterogeneity of results within the class of drugs, especially due to the class members that have smaller development programmes and would have fewer prospects to detect specific AEs of interest [48] Thus, the issue of size is more complex in meta-analysis of a class of drugs than for a single drug.

3.7 Multi-arm trials

Summary of main points:

▸ In a multi-arm clinical trial, there may be two or more intervention groups with one common control group. Alternatively, there may be more than one control group such as a placebo group and a standard treatment group.

▸ If multiple arms are not handled correctly, this will result in double counting of the control group, which will lead to bias in the meta-analysis because certain results are overrepresented.

▸ How to address the pair-wise comparisons when a multi-arm trial is included in meta-analysis should be determined on a case-by-case basis, according to the specific situation.

▶ In some situations it will be advisable to combine groups to create a single pair-wise comparison. However, combining a high-dose group and a low-dose group could dilute the effect of the high dose or inflate the effect of the low dose.

In a multi-arm clinical trial, there may be two or more intervention groups with one common control group. Alternatively, there may be more than one control group, such as a placebo group, and a standard treatment group. One common issue encountered is how to address the pair-wise comparisons when a multi-arm trial is included in meta-analysis.

Often, a multi-arm study is a three-armed parallel trial in which there are two interventions (intervention 1 and intervention 2) compared with a control. These might be a low-dose and high-dose arm of the experimental treatment. When each intervention group is entered into the analysis separately (e.g. if "low dose vs. placebo" and "high dose vs. placebo" are both included in the same meta-analysis), the control group will be counted twice. As such, a unit-of-analysis problem arises; it can result in studies receiving more weight than is appropriate. This problem is referred to as double counting of the control group and leads to bias in meta-analysis from certain results being overrepresented [104].

There is no single right answer regarding methods for including multi-arm trials in meta-analysis when more than two of the groups are relevant. The decision, therefore, should be determined on a case-by-case basis, depending on the specific situation. One possible method in many situations is to combine groups to create a single pair-wise comparison [6]. However, combining a high-dose group and a low-dose group could dilute the effect of the high dose or inflate the effect of the low dose. Methods that allow the inclusion of both dose groups separately (see below), might permit the assessment of a dose–response relationship.

There are different methods for combining various intervention groups, depending on the types of outcomes being assessed. When the main safety information studied is the number of patients with the event (or counts of events) and the total number of patients (or patient years) in each group, many publications report the original counts of events. Under such circumstances, avoidance of double counting can be achieved by combining the two groups and essentially treating them as a single group. This would be done by adding the original counts of events across the two dose groups and adding the total number of patients (or patient years) directly across the two dose groups [105]. Sometimes, the health outcome of interest in a safety study is a continuous variable, and the main safety data assessed are the total number of patients in each group, the mean of the outcome in each group, and the standard deviation in each group.

Under such circumstances, means and standard deviations from multiple intervention groups can be combined to recreate a combined treatment group across arms of the trial [6]. However, this approach may lead to incorrect conclusions about the data. For example, a certain multi-arm trial may have either two control groups consisting of a placebo and a standard treatment group, or more than two active control groups using different drugs. When the placebo and various standard treatments have different effects on study outcomes, bias would be introduced as a result of combining such groups to create a single pair-wise comparison. The problem is similar to the issue discussed above of combining across dose groups for the same experimental treatment. If the two different comparators (as with a low dose and a high dose) have different effects on the risk of the event under study, interpreting a result from the combined group would be challenging.

A further possibility in overcoming the unit-of-analysis error due to double counting is to account for the correlation between correlated comparisons from the same study in the analysis. Bayesian hierarchical models used for meta-analysis can incorporate correlated comparisons within the same studies. Gleser & Olkin [106] present a frequentist alternative.

The discussion of multi-arm trials also leads to another issue for consideration – i.e. determining if all groups of all studies should be considered eligible for the same meta-analysis. As a simple example, if the question of interest is the increased risk of cardiovascular events associated with a particular nonsteroidal anti-inflammatory drug (NSAID) as compared with placebo, and a trial compares that NSAID with both placebo and another NSAID, the appropriate choice might be to exclude the second NSAID from the analysis. If a class effect is being examined, that decision would not be appropriate. If it is necessary to assess the intervention drug separately against each comparator; each comparison would need to be addressed in a separate meta-analysis unless a mixed-treatment comparison is performed.

3.8 Risk of bias of the meta-analysis, individual study and overall

Summary of main points:

▶ RCTs are seldom designed and powered specifically to evaluate drug safety. Thus, aspects of design that do not affect the validity of the study for evaluating primary efficacy endpoints may still affect the validity of safety assessments.

▶ RCTs are often compromised by high rates of individual subjects withdrawing from the study prematurely, which may introduce attrition bias, particularly in trials of long-term follow-up.

▶ Occurrence of known drug-related AEs may unmask the assigned treatment and introduce bias, particularly in the absence of a pre-specified plan for the ascertainment and adjudication of AEs.

▶ Enrichment of RCT study populations, ordinarily intended to improve trial efficiency through improving patient participation and response and allowing estimation of long-term benefits of treatment, may actually result in underestimation of rates of drug-related AEs.

▶ Combining RCTs for different drugs within a drug class may be needed to investigate uncommon AEs, but the interpretability of summary estimates relies on the assumption that any increase in rate of a particular AE is similar within that class.

The quality of the information derived from meta-analysis clearly depends to a large extent on the validity of the included studies. This statement seems obvious, but has some subtle implications in the context of safety assessment. RCTs are seldom designed and powered specifically to evaluate drug safety. Thus, aspects of design that do not affect the validity of the study for evaluating primary efficacy endpoints may still affect the validity of safety assessments. Potential limitations might be exacerbated in the study of rare outcomes, which are often encountered in drug safety assessment. In some situations, randomization may not be completely successful, which could lead to persistent imbalance in important risk factors and thereby could have an impact on the validity of the relative risk estimates if only unadjusted estimates are used. Optimally, meta-analyses should be prospectively planned. However, the post-hoc nature of some meta-analyses introduces potential biases inherent to any retrospective observational studies [27, 107-110].

Several tools for assessing RCT "quality" have been proposed [111-113]. Olivo et al. reviewed scales used to evaluate the methodological quality of RCTs and concluded that most of the scales have not been properly developed and recommended against weighing trials by quality scores in meta-analyses [114]. Jüni and colleagues [115] showed that the relationship between study "quality" and study findings depends heavily on the measure of quality [116]. An increasingly popular view is that individual aspects of the trial design and conduct are more useful to examine as potential sources of bias than any arbitrarily-weighted summary score derived from the individual items [116, 117]. However, what constitutes a challenge in the evaluation of sources of bias is the paucity of information reported in published meta-analyses about various aspects of the component studies that could be pertinent to drug safety [48]. This section addresses some of the threats to validity and opportunities for bias in randomized trials that are included in meta-analyses as well as attempts to combine these trials.

3.8.1 Frailty of randomization resulting from premature trial discontinuation

In practice, RCTs are often compromised by high rates of individual subjects withdrawing from the study prematurely [118], which may introduce attrition bias. Attrition is particularly problematic in trials of long-term follow-up, because of the increased likelihood of patients dropping out of trials with the passage of time. For example, in meta-analysis examining the association between antidepressant drugs and suicidality among adolescents [9], the rate of discontinuation in trials ranged from 8% to 66%, with significant differences in discontinuation rates between comparison groups in several trials. Substantial trial discontinuation rates (up to 42%) were also noted among several trials in a meta-analysis examining the association between inhaled anticholinergics and the risk of major adverse cardiovascular events in patients with chronic obstructive pulmonary disease (COPD) [15]. Adjustment for imbalances in known and measured characteristics may be possible, but adjustment for imbalances in unmeasured characteristics is more challenging. Various methods have been proposed for assessing the sensitivity of observed associations to the possible effect of unobserved confounders [119-122]. When reasons for discontinuation are also related to the probability of developing the AE of interest, further bias can be introduced. For example, if patients with chest pain, who are at increased risk of subsequent myocardial infarction, withdraw prematurely (and, arguably, appropriately from a clinical perspective) from the drug group, the association between drug exposure and myocardial infarction may not be detected (i.e. the risk of myocardial infarction in the drug group is artificially reduced by the withdrawals). In another example, a study retrospectively reviewed mortality rates in a 6-month RCT in which an inhaled anticholinergic drug was shown to decrease COPD exacerbations. In this study, premature discontinuation of trial treatment occurred in 15% and 8% of the placebo and drug groups, respectively. Importantly, sicker patients (i.e. those with poorer lung function) on the inferior treatment (i.e. placebo) were more likely to discontinue the trial (i.e. the risk of mortality is artificially lowered in the placebo group by the withdrawals, making the drug group look worse) [123].

Controlling for the resulting imbalances across study groups is challenging, as reasons for trial discontinuation and information concerning health and vital status among patients who discontinued from a trial are typically not captured with sufficient granularity. It is important to remember that such bias can favour either treatment group. For example, hypothetically, in the trial of anticholinergic drugs, the sicker patients who experience symptom relief on active treatment, and who tend to remain in the trial longer than their counterparts in the placebo group, might also be at increased risk of AEs because of the increased severity of the underlying illness unrelated to drug exposure.

3.8.2   Unmasking of drug assignment

Failure of masking (blinding) may also compromise the validity of AE evaluations. In some situations, occurrence of known drug-related AEs may unmask the assigned treatment and introduce bias, particularly in absence of a pre-specified plan for the ascertainment and adjudication of AEs. This is a particular challenge when certain AEs are known to be associated with an entire class of drugs (e.g. sexual dysfunction with antidepressant drugs) [124].

Unmasking might lead to increased awareness and surveillance, ultimately leading to a higher probability of detection of other AEs among patients receiving the drug compared to placebo. Similarly, drug-related AEs may result in more frequent interaction with health-care providers. For instance, in the Women's Health Initiative study, blinding was prematurely broken due to occurrence and management of hormone replacement therapy (HRT)-associated vaginal bleeding for more women in the drug arm compared to placebo [125]. Other examples might include a drug that leads to urine discoloration and subsequently to an apparent increase in risk of urinary tract cancer that could be due entirely to surveillance (detection) bias. Similarly, a drug that leads to breast tenderness might lead to increased diagnostic testing for breast cancer and a subsequent apparent (but spurious) increase in risk of breast cancer.

Unmasking of drug assignment can also occur prior to randomization when those randomized sequences are not protected by adequate concealment of the allocation sequence from those involved in the enrolment and assignment of participants. Knowledge of the next assignment can cause selective enrolment of participants on the basis of risk factors. Failures to conceal allocation tend to overestimate beneficial results, and may also introduce an important bias related to drug safety.

3.8.3   Ascertainment of adverse events

A number of issues related to inconsistent ascertainment of AEs can also compromise safety assessments. For example, the lack of an *a priori* AE definition, or tools specifically designed to ascertain a specific AE, can be particularly problematic. It is not always possible to anticipate which AEs will be important, and it may not be feasible to produce specific *a priori* definitions for all possible AEs, so it becomes very important to do periodic assessments of safety data during development (not just at the end of Phase III), so as to be able to modify data collection for subsequent trials. However, if one is considering changing the method of data collection of AEs, the impact on future meta-analyses should also be considered. For example, separate analyses might be planned and performed for studies before and after the change in method of AE collection. That separation could, in turn, have consequences. If the post-change data are considered *a priori* to be more valid and therefore become the primary analysis, then that could limit the statistical power to detect an increase in risk, unless the size of the increase in risk is also greater due perhaps to increased specificity of the AE definition.

Comparisons across trials are made difficult by differences across trials in the completeness of clinical narratives. Furthermore, not all AEs are documented in RCT reports that are prepared for non-regulatory purposes or in publications (a form of reporting bias). Published trial reports are sometimes silent on AEs [126], highlighting the importance of contacting original investigators, if feasible, to obtain additional relevant information from trials that may not have been included in the original trial report or publication [127]. Meta-analyses evaluating the association between anticholinergic and cardiovascular events [15] excluded trials that were silent on the cardiovascular AE of interest, presumably because the rates were low, resulting in exclusion of approximately two-thirds of available trials. Exclusion of a large number of trials is likely to have biased the meta-analysis results, if the event rates were not balanced in the omitted trials. The suggested increase in risk of cardiovascular events observed in the meta-analysis was later refuted by a large, long-term, placebo-controlled randomized clinical trial [128]. (Note: A related issue, covered in section 4.2, is the handling of studies that properly assessed and reported AEs, and explicitly report no events occurring in either treatment group.)

Enrichment of RCT study populations, ordinarily intended to improve trial efficiency through improving patient participation and response, can also influence the interpretation of drug safety data from RCTs. For example, in the randomized withdrawal design, patients who do not respond to or tolerate the drug during the initial open stabilization period are typically excluded from the trial. Whereas this strategy may enhance trial efficiency, and allows estimation of long-term benefits of treatment, it may result in underestimation of rates of drug-related AEs [129]. In an antidepressant trial, only 280 of the 533 initially enrolled patients who responded to the drug (and presumably tolerated it) were subsequently randomized during the double-blind treatment phase. Although rates of discontinuation due to AEs were nearly identical for drug and placebo groups during the double-blind treatment phase, 61 (24%) patients discontinued trial participation due to development of AEs during the initial phase that entailed being exposed to the drug. However, the rate of AEs during the phase prior to randomization, although informative, is often not considered in a drug's safety evaluation profile [130]. Similarly, AE underestimation can occur with cross-over designs when patients cross over to the comparison treatment arm, as patients who did not tolerate the drug in the first phase might be likely to drop out and be unavailable to participate in the second phase of the trial.

3.8.4 Capture of individual trials

A frequent concern about meta-analyses is the possibility of publication bias – i.e. the selective publication of studies based on the nature of their findings. When entire studies are not published, there might be a major threat to the validity of meta-analyses attempting to evaluate the totality of available evidence [131].

Funnel plots can be used to check for asymmetry in distribution of study results in a meta-analysis that may be indicative of publication bias [132]. A funnel plot is a simple scatter plot of the intervention effect estimates from individual studies against some measure of each study's size or precision. In the absence of bias the plot should approximately resemble a symmetrical funnel, as illustrated in Figure 3.1. The points in this graph plot the treatment effect (presented as odds ratio on the horizontal axis) against a measure of study size (presented as the standard error of log odds ratio on the vertical axis) for each single trial. Smaller trials tend to have larger standard errors and hence these appear towards the bottom of the graph. However, if there is a bias, such as when smaller studies without statistically significant effects (shown as open circles in Figure 3.1) remain unpublished, this will lead to an asymmetrical appearance of the funnel plot with a gap in a bottom corner of the graph.

Figure 3.1 Hypothetical funnel plots: symmetrical plot in the absence of bias

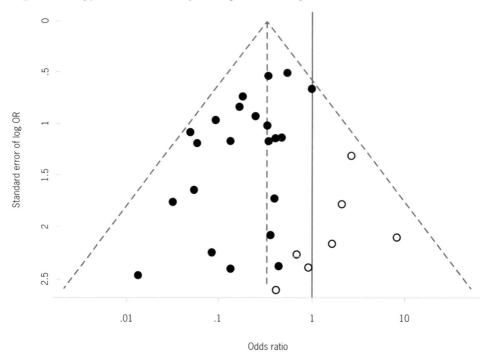

Source: Figure 10.4.a Cochrane Handbook for Systematic Reviews of Interventions [6]. Used with permission of the publishers.

Figure 3.2 below provides an example which provides the results of 15 trials which investigated the effect of magnesium on mortality following a myocardial infarction [133]. In this meta-analysis, most of the smaller trials provide a reduced mortality risk which could not be confirmed by the subsequent larger trials, resulting in a strong asymmetric funnel plot. It is worth noting that an asymmetrical funnel plot should not be equated automatically with publication bias because asymmetry could also be caused by other factors, such as differences in methodological quality. It is imperative to distinguish the different possible reasons for funnel plot asymmetry in interpreting funnel plots.

Figure 3.2 Asymmetrical plot in the presence of bias.

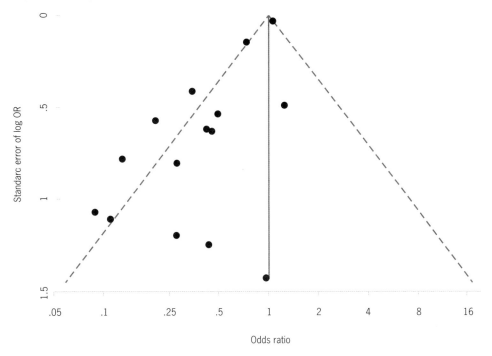

Source: Sterne & Harbord. Funnel plots in meta-analysis. Stata Journal, 2004, Figure 2, p.131 [133]. Used with permission of the publishers.

Recent requirements to register RCTs on clinicaltrials.gov might reduce the impact of selective reporting at the study level by making more data available for meta-analysis [134]. Similarly, the policy announced by industry organizations in Europe and the USA (http://phrma.org/sites/default/files/pdf/PhRMAPrinciplesForResponsibleClinicalTrialDataSharing.pdf), which commits sponsors to making full regulatory study reports and even individual participant data available to scientists who request it, is intended to reduce the possibility of publication bias, and would allow analyses of otherwise unreported endpoints (as well as potentially encouraging more complete reporting in the first place).

As an example of the potential consequences of publication bias, a concern about a potential increase in mortality associated with the use of cefepime was raised with the publication of a meta-analysis; however, the lack of inclusion of all trials substantively altered the findings [135]. In order to investigate this signal, the US FDA undertook a year-long effort in which findings from all published and unpublished cefepime clinical trials were examined [10]. The FDA analysis included 88 trials compared with 57 trials in the original meta-analysis. The increase in mortality reported by the initial meta-analysis was not confirmed in the larger and more detailed meta-analysis conducted by the FDA.

In contrast, the problem of multiple counting of trials/participants [104] has received less attention, although several examples can be found in the literature, including articles in leading medical journals [15, 136]. It may therefore be important to communicate with clinical trialists to ensure that different publications actually reflect distinct study populations.

3.8.5 Suitability of trials for integration

Integration of data across trials is appropriate when the studies are clinically "similar", i.e. they are addressing the "same" clinical question, and the treatment effect is expected to be relatively similar across RCTs. However, defining terms like "similar" and "the same clinical question" can be challenging. Differences in trial design, protocol nuances or implementation, drug indication, inclusion and exclusion criteria, duration and dose of treatment, and case ascertainment practices for AEs might lead to differences in findings across studies and make summary estimates difficult to interpret. As mentioned in section 3.5.1, the mere fact that several studies have the similar initial protocol might not guarantee the studies' similarity. The actual execution of the protocols might be different from one study to another [48]. Combining RCTs for different drugs within a drug class may be needed to investigate uncommon AEs [9], but the interpretability of summary estimates relies on the assumption that any increase in rate of a particular AE is similar within that class. That assumption may not be valid and will often be difficult to verify or refute, especially when events are uncommon. Furthermore, when meta-analysts integrate trials that were conducted over many years [9], changes in medical practice resulting from the availability of improved therapies or new technology may contribute additional variability across trials.

3.8.6 Unit of analysis issues

The Cochrane Handbook provides a useful summary of unit-of-analysis issues, reproduced below, and contains a more detailed list of situations in which unit-of-analysis issues commonly arise, together with directions to relevant discussions elsewhere in the Handbook [6].

> An important principle concerning the clinical trials incorporated into a meta-analysis is that the level of analysis must align with the level at which randomization occurred. In practice, this often (but not always) means that the number of observations in the analysis should match the number of "units" that were randomized. More generally, adjustments for so-called "design effects" should be applied in the analysis. These can result in a kind of effective sample size that falls between the number of units randomized and the total number of individuals within those units.

> In a simple parallel group design, for example, individuals are randomized to one of two intervention groups, and a single measurement for each outcome from each participant is collected and analysed. However, the actual randomization approach can vary in ways that are important to consider. Authors should consider whether in each study:

> 1. groups of individuals were randomized collectively to the same intervention (i.e. cluster-randomized trials);

> 2. more than one intervention is applied (in random order) to each individual (e.g. in a cross-over trial, or simultaneous treatment of multiple sites on each individual); or

> 3. even with a single intervention applied to each individual, there are multiple observations for the same outcome (e.g. repeated measurements, recurring events, measurements on different body parts).

3.9 Access to individual participant data, summary-level data, or both

Summary of main points:

▶ Although many meta-analyses, traditionally, have been based on summary-level data - usually meaning published data there is increasing interest in the use of IPD.

▶ Advantages of using IPD in the context of a meta-analysis include the ability to do the following:

— Map all data to a common set of definitions, thereby increasing consistency of terminology across trials (e.g. standardizing the level of haemoglobin at which "anaemia" is defined).

— Use composite variables to define outcomes on the basis of a combination of variables, each of which defines a specific event, but that collectively may indicate a common physiological mechanism. As an example, an AE (e.g. appetite suppression) might be defined as a combination of weight loss or appetite reduction.

— Analyse time-to-event, which would not be easily accomplished using summary-level data when those data appear in the form of simple proportions.

— Estimate treatment effects in subgroups of participants defined by participant-level (as opposed to summary-level) characteristics.

— Adjust for imbalances between comparator groups (e.g. by taking into consideration various demographics and comorbidities at the individual participant level).

▷ Methods have been developed for situations in which a combination of summary-level data and IPD are available.

▷ Meta-analysis is considered by some to represent an observational design, such that outcomes, inferences and interpretations should be described as associations rather than reported using causal terms.

Although many published meta-analyses are based only on summary-level data, there are potential advantages of using IPD. In reality, most of the important analytical principles (e.g. stratification by study) apply to both patient-level and summary-level analytical approaches.

Analyses that can be done in a summary-level data meta-analysis can also be done with an IPD meta-analysis, but the converse is not true. Advantages of IPD are described below. Given those advantages, it would be reasonable to ask why IPD are not always utilized during drug development when the sponsor is likely to have access to all of the relevant studies and the associated IPD. There are at least two important reasons. First, the integration that is required to create the analytical database is labour intensive, especially if done in retrospect. Moreover, the integration is even more challenging and labour intensive when a class of drug effects is of interest with respect to a safety issue and therefore data have to come from multiple sponsors, who may have used different definitions of AEs or different durations of follow-up. The second reason is that sometimes IPD may not be available for some studies of interest, even to the sponsor that markets the drug. For example, studies of a new indication for an existing drug may have been conducted by an academic cooperative group that does not share patient-level data, or the drug of interest may have been included as an active control by another sponsor. Importantly, one should consider when the considerable extra effort required to use IPD is valuable. In some situations, such as when there is no need to re-evaluate any aspects of individual-level data (e.g. calculating time-to-event, investigating differential discontinuation between the drug and comparator groups, or recoding AEs), and when the question being addressed does not involve subgroups defined by patient characteristics, a summary-level data meta-analysis will give the same answer as the corresponding IPD meta-analysis [137].

Importantly, many of the limitations to meta-analysis that apply to summary-level data meta-analysis also apply to IPD. As the accompanying editorial to the PRISMA-IPD reporting guidance notes, "…the increasing interest in data sharing is likely to lead to a proliferation of IPD meta-analyses, so this study design will be increasingly relevant to authors and readers" [19]. It is also of interest that, in a commentary in the Journal of the American Medical Association (JAMA) co-authored by one of the JAMA editors, the authors note, "Accordingly, JAMA considers meta-analysis to represent an observational design, such that outcomes, inferences, and interpretations should be described as associations rather than reported using causal terms such as 'size of effect', as suggested by the PRISMA-IPD statement" [25].

3.9.1 Advantages of individual participant-level data

Changes in data standards are to be expected during the course of the development of any drug. As a simple example, consider changes and updates to coding systems and dictionaries. When AE information is reported on the basis of a new dictionary version (e.g. of the Medical Dictionary for Regulatory Activities, or MedDRA) [80], the same term can be mapped to a different preferred term and/or differences at higher levels of the hierarchy may occur. Access to IPD allows mapping all data to a common version of MedDRA and, therefore, will increase consistency of terminology and definitions across trials. Access to IPD generally allows the creation of variables that are common to all studies. For example, age categories for stratification of results may have been defined using different category boundaries, or different threshold haemoglobin values may have been used to define "anaemia". In such situations, access to patient-level data allows standardization across trials that would not have been possible based on summary-level data alone. Definitions of censoring events may also be standardized using IPD, again not an option when limited to summary-level data.

Patient-level data permit using composite variables to define outcomes based on combination of variables, each of which defines a specific event but that collectively may indicate a common physiological mechanism. As an example, an AE might be defined as a combination of weight loss or appetite reduction. One might also be able to check on concordance of different measures of the same underlying problem (e.g. weight loss as an AE or a decrease in measured body weight beyond a specified threshold). In addition, post hoc analyses of outcomes that require adjudication can sometimes be performed, as in the case of suicide event grading according to the Columbia Classification Algorithm of Suicide Assessment (C-CASA criteria) [82]. Such post hoc adjudication can play an important role in standardizing definitions and how they are operationalized across studies, thereby making the treatment effects more comparable (although not necessarily more similar) across studies.

Patient-level data also permit analysing time-to-event, which would not be easily accomplished using summary-level data when those data appear in the form of simple proportions. With patient-level data, Kaplan-Meier time-to-event graphs can help identify events with changing hazard rates over time (e.g. there could be a separation in acute events related to initial exposure that goes away with longer follow-up), or events that have a latent induction period (e.g. cancer). With IPD, some of the important assumptions for survival analysis can be checked. The dependence of the hazard ratio on time (e.g. to check whether the hazard ratio is constant over time) can and should be examined using the IPD. This could be estimated by either a time by treatment interaction in the Cox model, a logrank analysis within discrete units of time over T and/or by inspection of a Kaplan-Meier curve. (Note though that a Kaplan-Meier curve of more than one study combined can be misleading. It is important to check the studies one at a time.) These study-specific interactions and variances can be used to calculate a summary measure of interaction over all studies. It is possible, in a case where a drug is known to increase the risk of an event, that the interactions themselves could be the primary reason for the meta-analysis – i.e. the interest is in understanding how long after the start of exposure the risk increases or decreases.

An important advantage of IPD is the ability to estimate effects for subgroups of patients defined by subject-level characteristics. As an example, consider an analysis by Szczech and colleagues, in which the authors were able to examine the specific effects of induction therapy (essentially, prophylactic treatment to prevent rejection of transplanted kidneys) in subgroups of patients at high risk for kidney transplant failure [138]. This is not strictly a "safety" question, but the example illustrates the potential importance of the flexibility provided by access to patient-level data. The authors were able to detect an interaction between treatment and a patient-level characteristic that could not be identified with only summary-level data. Specifically, one covariate of interest was the panel reactive antibody level (PRA), an indicator of immune system sensitization.

After two years of follow-up, the authors showed that the effect of induction therapy differed in sensitized and non-sensitized patients ($P = 0.03$ for the interaction) using IPD. This interaction was still significant at five years of follow-up. In contrast, this interaction was not consistently demonstrated in analyses performed with summary-level data, using the "percent of sensitized patients" as a study-level characteristic, and regressing "treatment effect" against the study-level covariate [139]. One could argue that it would be important to confirm such subgroup results in an independent data set; if confirmed, these results could mean that induction therapy could be targeted to the group in which it is highly effective, while avoiding needless treatment and potential toxicity in other patients.

Use of summary-level data for detecting subgroup effects has other limitations. Lambert and colleagues, for instance, show that analyses based on summary-level data often have low statistical power to detect interactions (also known as effect modification) [140]. Similarly, Schmid and colleagues showed that subgroup differences of interest were detected by patient-level analyses but not by summary-level analyses [141]. In one analysis, treatment effects were homogeneous across studies and therefore meta-regression identified no interactions, despite the existence of interactions within studies that were evident using patient-level data. Nonetheless, an important point is that having access only to summary-level data does not rule out exploration of treatment-effect modifiers. Examining potential sources of heterogeneity of study findings, such as dose, duration or other study-level factors, can still shed light on important clinical questions.

A concept related to subgroup analyses is that of using the IPD to evaluate risk factors for AEs. This could be extremely valuable in defining groups of patients who are at high risk of an event, which would affect the estimated treatment effect in absolute terms, even if there is no interaction on the relative risk scale. This absolute increase would affect the benefit-risk assessment. For example, if a particular subgroup of patients with non-valvular atrial fibrillation is at high risk of a bleeding event related to an anticoagulant, that risk would need to be considered in evaluating the trade-off against reduction in risk of stroke, even if there were no subgroup by treatment interaction on the relative scale. More discussions on subgroup analyses using the IPD can be found in section 4.8.1.

In some situations, one might have access to IPD in some, but not all, studies. Riley & Steyerberg present meta-analysis models that permit synthesis of observed event-risks across studies, while accounting for the within-study association between participant-level covariates and event probabilities [69]. The models are adapted for situations where studies provide a mixture of IPD and summary-level data. They note that it is often essential to model within-study associations and separate them from across-study associations in order to account for potential ecological bias and study-level confounding.

3.10 Specific issues in meta-analysis of observational studies

Summary of main points:

▶ The risk of bias is high in individual observational studies and may be exacerbated when they are combined.

▶ Meta-analysis of observational studies may be considered for one or more of the following purposes:

— to decide whether a randomized trial is necessary or to inform the design of a new trial by evaluation of the weaknesses of available observational studies;

— to provide evidence of the effects of interventions that cannot be randomized, or of outcomes that are extremely unlikely to be studied in randomized trials (such as long-term and rare outcomes); and/or

— to study the effects in patient groups not customarily studied in randomized trials (such as children, pregnant women and older patients).

▶ Combining effect estimates from observational studies with effect estimates from randomized trials in a single analysis is not recommended.

▶ Combining observational studies that have dissimilar study design features may be an important source of heterogeneity and caution in combining them must be exercised.

3.10.1 Background

This report has targeted the possibly more difficult area of looking at unintended effects – the harms of medicines and other medical interventions. Even combining all the randomized evidence for some issues may not provide clear answers. This will basically be because the numbers of harmful events may still be too small in the population of interest. Recruitment to trials may underrepresent or exclude vulnerable patient groups (e.g. older persons, patients with multiple comorbidities, children, and women of child-bearing age). It may be that the length of follow-up is inadequate; the population of interest has been too small or not studied at all. Many trials may be adequately powered to study surrogate outcomes but too small to study clinical outcomes. Other sources of evidence may then be necessary to answer some questions of interest [142]. Observational studies are defined here as any quantitative study estimating the effectiveness or safety of an intervention (benefit or harm) in which treatment allocation occurs in the course of usual treatment decisions.

There are many types of observational study and they include between-person comparisons (cohort or case-control-type designs) and within-person comparisons (self-controlled designs) [143]. A complete description of possible study designs is beyond the scope of this report, but the interested reader is referred to standard textbooks on epidemiology and pharmacoepidemiology for further reading [144, 145]. A framework for assessing designs has been set out very clearly by Pearce [146].

The Cochrane Collaboration has in recent years, particularly through its Adverse Effects Methods Group (AEMG), acknowledged that observational data may be important in some instances [87, 147]. The empirical evidence is that meta-analyses of randomized and observational data give similar results when looking at adverse effects [148]. An earlier study suggested that observational studies can give lower estimates of relative effects [149]. The design of observational studies often excludes those with a known high risk of the event of interest, particularly a previous history of that event, but in clinical practice such patients may well be treated. This means that the absolute rate of ADRs may be underestimated. This section covers some of the more technical or statistical aspects, but some issues of principle are addressed first.

3.10.2 Principles

Randomized evidence can have a variety of biases, but there is no doubt that data from non-randomized studies can have all the biases found in randomized trials and a great many other biases in addition. The main biases relate to the fact that those treated with one drug are very different from those who are not treated and may well be different from those given another drug for the same condition. "Confounding by indication" (a form of channelling bias) can occur when the reason for prescription is associated with both the treatment and the outcome of interest. For example, proton pump inhibitors are used in the management of upper gastrointestinal bleeding and also in the treatment of heartburn. Randomized trials have demonstrated the efficacy of these drugs for this indication. In attempting to study the association between use of proton pump inhibitors and upper gastrointestinal bleeding, one might see an apparently paradoxical increase in risk associated with drug exposure. This could result from the increased frequency of use of these drugs for the treatment of symptoms that occur prior to the bleeding diagnosis. Since exposure to a particular drug is determined not by random allocation but by circumstances that could be related to the outcome of interest, observed drug-outcome relationships may be systematically overestimated or underestimated. For instance, physicians prescribe novel therapies to patients who have failed existing therapies or have more severe disease, increasing the likelihood of finding that the novel therapy produces a greater rate of AEs or worsening outcome when those events might be unrelated to treatment. The way in which the treated and comparison groups differ will never be known completely. Even where some knowledge of differences is available, adjustment for those differences will also never be perfect.

Observational studies have even greater potential for methodological diversity than RCTs, through variation in design and execution. Particular concerns arise with respect to differences between people in different intervention groups (selection bias) and studies that do not explicitly report having had a protocol and having planned the analysis of the particular question of interest (reporting bias). One issue is that, without a protocol, selective reporting of results of many analyses may occur. There is always potential for bias in the results of the observational studies; therefore any systematic review or meta analysis of them must consider the risk of bias, including both its likely direction and its magnitude in individual studies. The risk of bias is already high in individual observational studies and may be exacerbated when they are combined. A recent review of available assessment tools for evaluating epidemiological studies showed that the majority of tools did not include critical assessment elements that are specifically relevant to drug safety studies [150]. For meta-analyses of observational studies it is important to consider: (a) design weaknesses; (b) a careful assessment of risk of bias, in the conduct of individual studies; and (c) the potential for reporting biases, including selective reporting of outcomes. There is a "Risk of Bias" assessment tool, developed by persons involved in the Cochrane Collaboration, that mirrors a similar tool for randomized studies (see https://sites.google.com/site/riskofbiastool/).

In spite of these reservations, meta-analysis of observational studies may be considered for one or more of the following purposes:

▶ to decide whether a randomized trial is necessary or to inform the design of a new trial by evaluation of the weaknesses of available observational studies;

▶ to provide evidence of the effects of interventions that should not be randomized (e.g. because of ethical concerns, or outcomes that are extremely unlikely to be studied in randomized trials such as long-term and rare outcomes; and/or

▶ to study the effects in patient groups not customarily studied in randomized trials (such as children, pregnant women and older patients) because of ethical or other considerations.

A clear consequence of this is that the treatment of randomized and non-randomized evidence as equivalent (exchangeable) in a single analysis is a mistake; combination of data must distinguish between them. Some efforts have been made, particularly in a Bayesian paradigm, to combine evidence from both sources in a single analysis, but the methods for doing this are not yet widely agreed.

The major message is that uncertainty in treatment effects is not only dependent on sampling variation but on many other factors. In fact, the sampling variation may be extremely small because observational data may have very large numbers of patients and events, and standard CIs do not cover the uncertainty in effect in the same way as a CI from a randomized trial.

3.10.3 Questions about observational study data validity

It is important to consider questions of validity of observational study data. This inquiry is even more important with observational studies than it is with randomized trials.

How are studies selected?

This text obviously applies to RCTs, but with observational studies there is a greater chance of publication bias. With RCTs, many drug trials in the early life history of a drug are under the control of, or well known to, the sponsor making the drug and the regulatory authorities. Even if this is not the case, in many instances and especially in the future it will apply to all as the RCTs will have been registered with a protocol either at Clinicaltrials.gov or a similar registry often related to regulatory requirements. In contrast, observational studies will often not be under the control of, or even known to, the relevant drug sponsor or regulatory authorities and will have been conducted some time after marketing. The protocol may not have been registered, although registration is increasing in frequency, especially through the use of the publicly accessible E-Register of Studies maintained by the *European Network of Centres for Pharmacoepidemiology and Pharmacovigilance* (ENCePP) [151] registry, and one industry group has advocated registration of observational studies whenever there is a predefined question [152]. The consequence of this situation is that unbiased selection of studies may be very difficult. It will rarely be possible to have prospective specification of observational studies to be included in a future meta-analysis.

In most instances, the results will be known at the time when an observational study is considered for inclusion, thereby increasing the potential for bias. The large size of observational studies tempts the investigators to carry out many subgroup analyses. In RCTs the interpretation of subgroups is difficult, but in observational studies the potential for vast numbers of analyses, which are not pre-specified, is enormous. Combining these studies, especially their subgroups, is then problematic.

Has confounding been dealt with adequately in each study?

Assessment of potential for bias is necessary in meta-analysis of RCTs, and the Cochrane "Risk of Bias" tool is one way of doing this [62]. The development of a similar tool for observational studies has been noted above, and there is a need for very careful assessment, especially of "confounding by indication", which is a form of channelling bias. Such assessments are subjective so the results must be treated with caution. The Strengthening the Reporting of Observational Studies in Epidemiology (STROBE) guidelines may be used to ensure that reporting of the observational studies has been done well [153]. There should usually be tables with the important risk factors, not only giving their distribution between treated and comparison groups, but also showing their association with the outcome of interest.

Are studies likely to be at low risk of bias?

RCTs can vary in terms of their risk of bias, but the range of risk of bias in observational studies is very much greater. Judgement on suitability of studies for inclusion in a meta-analysis should be driven by how much potential for bias exist in a given study. As mentioned earlier, a recent review of available assessment tools for evaluating epidemiologic studies showed that the majority of tools did not include critical assessment elements that are specifically relevant to drug safety studies [150]. Frequently the data were collected for other purposes, such as routine electronic health records, so the definition of terms may not be standardized. The use of standard methodologies to classify terms does not mean the data using such a classification are as well-defined as might be implied. There will be much missing data, and the methods used to allow for this may need to be examined carefully. Complete case analysis is not always unbiased.

These limitations may apply both to outcome variables as well as to risk factor covariates. The definition and reliability of exposures may have similar limitations and frequently rely on prescription data, but even if dispensing data are available this does not mean that participants were actually exposed. There are time-related biases that can occur and a high-quality study will explore the potential for these biases and attempt to minimize them.

How consistent are they?

It is vital to examine the heterogeneity of the studies. Investigation of reasons for this variability will be more important than simply carrying out significance tests.

Could a consistent bias across all studies explain the results?

This requires a lot of thought. It may be more relevant when observational studies attempt to look at benefits or other intended effects. Studies of unintended effects may be less likely to have consistent biases, but the possibility cannot be neglected.

Are the individual data available?

There have been cases of individual data being made available through a collaboration. An important example was the hormonal factors in breast cancer collaboration. Two major topics were studied and two papers published on hormonal contraceptives and on hormone (replacement) therapy [34, 154].

These studies were very useful in being able to look at effects related to factors not necessarily reported in the primary study reports but where the relevant data had been collected. An example would be "age at menopause" which seemed to be more important than age itself in affecting risk of breast cancer.

3.10.4 Conclusions on meta-analysis of observational data

If randomized data exist to answer the precise question of interest, it is best to rely on them. We do not recommend that effect estimates from observational studies be combined with effect estimates from randomized trials in a single analysis. Furthermore, in general, combining observational studies that have dissimilar study design features may be an important source of heterogeneity, and caution in combining them must be exercised. These design features may be good candidates for subgroup and/or sensitivity analyses.

When combining data across observational studies using meta-analysis, it is usually appropriate to analyse adjusted, rather than unadjusted, effect estimates – i.e. analyses that attempt to control for confounding if available. This may require authors to choose between alternative adjusted estimates reported for one study. Nonetheless, using adjusted effect estimates will not overcome the problem of residual confounding that is encountered in some studies that do not have information on all pertinent confounders. The source of residual confounding can differ between studies, in effect leading to estimates adjusted for a different subsets of confounders.

Where effects are very rare, it is possible that meta-analysis can be helpful, but the problem that uncertainty and variability in estimates from non-randomized data is not completely captured in ordinary CIs is not easily overcome.

As a related issue, meta-analyses of spontaneous postmarketing suspected adverse drug reaction reports (e.g. Adverse Event Reporting System) should be avoided. The most useful role of the information obtained from spontaneous postmarketing reports is to define a safety question of interest. These analyses are not appropriate for inclusion in any quantitative assessment of an overall effect.

In conclusion, observational studies and their systematic reviews are important in drug safety evaluation, but they require advanced methodological knowledge and cautious interpretation.

3.11 Network meta-analysis

When comparisons between different active treatments need to be made, it is often the case that few or no trials have made direct treatment comparisons. Nevertheless, each treatment may have been compared with placebo in multiple trials, and so it is possible to examine indirect comparisons. The assumptions required to do this make it advisable to treat indirect comparisons with greater caution than direct comparisons. However ,it may be the case that a new treatment is expected to be better than an old one and "novelty bias" may occur [155]. Additionally, all the caveats in this report that pertain to direct meta-analyses apply to, and may even be exacerbated in, network meta-analyses.

Several issues relate to the need to compare active treatments against each other. It may be that comparisons of interest may be estimated only through indirect comparison, as illustrated in Figure 3.3.

Figure 3.3 A connected network of randomized controlled trials to allow for indirect comparison meta-analysis

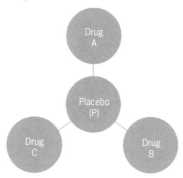

Source: Created by CIOMS X (2016).

In Figure 3.3, each of the three drugs has been compared to placebo in clinical trials, but none of the three drugs has been directly compared to each other. This assumes that there are at least three trials; A-P, B-P, C-P. In a meta-analysis, there may be multiple trials for each of these comparisons. In this situation, if the assumptions of the analysis are met, each of the drugs could be compared with each of the others, retaining the randomization, by virtue of the fact that all have a placebo comparator.

The basic principles of the analysis in such a situation are fairly intuitive [156]. In the simplest form, a comparison of Drug A with Drug B, assuming these are statistically independent trials, essentially involves taking the odds ratio for A vs. placebo and for B vs. placebo and taking their ratio. If the two trials are statistically independent, estimating a CI is straightforward in this simple situation.

There are several assumptions that are required for such an approach to yield valid results. Assessing heterogeneity of effects for a given pair-wise comparison of treatments is essential, as it would be for any meta-analysis. Perhaps the most challenging assumption to meet is that the study designs and populations are similar in a particular way. If there is a factor, such as severity of disease, that modifies the effect of one or more of the treatments, and the distribution of that factor differs across studies, then the comparison will not be valid. This applies, for example, if it is known (and it may not be known in advance of the analysis) that the treatment effect for the drugs in the comparison is larger for participants with more severe disease than for participants with less severe disease. A trial of Drug A that enrols mostly severe participants will tend to produce a larger treatment effect estimate than a trial of Drug A vs. placebo that enrols mostly non-severe participants. When both trials study Drug A, the difference in effect sizes might reasonably be attributed to disease severity. If the second trial involves a comparison of Drug B vs. placebo, it is less clear whether any difference in effect sizes is due to the different drug or the different disease severity, particularly if we do not anticipate the modification of treatment effect by disease severity. Factors that play this role need not be population characteristics; they could be study design elements (e.g. blinded vs. unblinded assessment of a subjective outcome measure). It is also worth noting that differences in participant characteristics that do not modify the effect of treatment do not cause this particular problem.

The next situation may be that there are at least some direct comparisons, say A-B and B-C. Again there may be multiple trials for these comparisons. This then allows for both direct and indirect comparisons to be made. This is referred to as "mixed treatment comparison". There is then a question of whether the different comparisons are "consistent" with each other – i.e. whether the direct comparisons and indirect comparisons of the same two treatments give similar results. There is some literature on the general problem with some suggestions for solutions around the inconsistency or "incoherence" of the comparisons [157-160].

The data that are available may be just the study summary results, or it may be that individual study participant data are available. A fairly recent example, where IPD were used where available, studied gastrointestinal and cardiovascular effects of non-steroidal anti-inflammatory drugs (NSAIDs) [161]. This paper looked at these two adverse effects of NSAIDs but simply used the Peto method for individual trials (based either on individual or summary data according to which was available) and averaged the effects across direct and indirect comparisons, using inverse variance methods. There was no estimate of inconsistency in the network as a whole or for particular comparisons, but estimates of the heterogeneity of the results for each comparison were obtained. Bayesian methods are often used in carrying out such analyses, and the whole field is very active in finding new methods.

Some effort is also being applied in using observational data in networks. Because of the complexity of the methods and because indirect comparisons are no longer randomized comparisons in the way that direct comparisons are, general guidance cannot yet be given on the best ways to carry out such analyses. Interpretation must be done with caution, especially where indirect comparisons are the majority of the data or the studies themselves are observational.

A relatively recent paper that covers many of the issues at a non-technical level is by Mills et al. [162]. Furthermore, Cochrane has put much effort into adapting network meta-analysis methodology and provides helpful material under the link http://cmimg.cochrane.org/.

References Chapter 3

6. Higgins JPT, Green S, eds. Cochrane Handbook for Systematic Reviews of Interventions Version 5.1.0 [updated March 2011]. 2011, The Cochrane Collaboration. http://handbook.cochrane.org/.

8. U.S. Food and Drug Administration. Guidance for industry: Diabetes mellitus-evaluating cardiovascular risk in new antidiabetic therapies to treat Type 2 diabetes. 2008. http://www.fda.gov/downloads/Drugs/GuidanceComplianceRegulatoryInformation/Guidances/UCM071627.pdf.

9. Hammad TA, Laughren T, Racoosin J. Suicidality in pediatric patients treated with antidepressant drugs. Arch Gen Psychiatry, 2006, 63(3): 332-339.

10. Kim PW, Wu YT, Cooper C, Rochester G, Valappil T, Wang Y, Kornegay C, Nambiar S. Meta-analysis of a possible signal of increased mortality associated with cefepime use. Clin Infect Dis, 2010, 51(4): 381-389.

15. Singh S, Loke YK, Furberg CD. Inhaled anticholinergics and risk of major adverse cardiovascular events in patients with chronic obstructive pulmonary disease: a systematic review and meta-analysis. JAMA, 2008, 300(12): 1439-1450.

19. Stewart LA, Clarke M, Rovers M, Riley RD, Simmonds M, Stewart G, Tierney JF, Group P-ID. Preferred Reporting Items for Systematic Review and Meta-Analyses of individual participant data: the PRISMA-IPD Statement. JAMA, 2015, 313(16): 1657-1665.

25. Berlin JA, Golub RM. Meta-analysis as evidence: building a better pyramid. JAMA, 2014, 312(6): 603-606.

27. Shapiro S. Meta-analysis/Shmeta-analysis. Am J Epidemiol, 1994, 140(9): 771-778.

34. Collaborative Group on Hormonal Factors in Breast Cancer. Breast cancer and hormonal contraceptives: collaborative reanalysis of individual data on 53 297 women with breast cancer and 100 239 women without breast cancer from 54 epidemiological studies. Lancet, 1996, 347(9017): 1713-1727.

47. Hammad TA, Neyarapally GA, Iyasu S, Staffa JA, Dal Pan G. The future of population-based postmarket drug risk assessment: a regulator's perspective. Clin Pharmacol Ther, 2013, 94(3): 349-358.

48. Hammad TA, Pinheiro SP, Neyarapally GA. Secondary use of randomized controlled trials to evaluate drug safety: a review of methodological considerations. Clin Trials, 2011, 8(5): 559-570.

59. CIOMS Working Group VI. Management of Safety Information from Clinical Trials. 2005, Geneva: Council for International Organizations of Medical Sciences.

60. Crowe BJ, Xia HA, Berlin JA, Watson DJ, Shi H, Lin SL, Kuebler J, Schriver RC, Santanello NC, Rochester G, Porter JB, Oster M, Mehrotra DV, Li Z, King EC, Harpur ES, Hall DB. Recommendations for safety planning, data collection, evaluation and reporting during drug, biologic and vaccine development: a report of the safety planning, evaluation, and reporting team. Clin Trials, 2009, 6(5): 430-440.

62. Higgins JP, Altman DG, Gotzsche PC, Juni P, Moher D, Oxman AD, Savovic J, Schulz KF, Weeks L, Sterne JA, Cochrane Bias Methods G, Cochrane Statistical Methods G. The Cochrane Collaboration's tool for assessing risk of bias in randomised trials. BMJ, 2011, 343: d5928.

67. University of York. PROSPERO, an international database of prospectively registered systematic reviews in health and social care. 2011, PROSPERO was launched by the NIHR on 22 February 2011 at U of York's Centre for Reviews and Dissemination. http://www.crd.york.ac.uk/prospero/search.asp.

68. Riley RD, Lambert PC, Staessen JA, Wang J, Gueyffier F, Thijs L, Boutitie F. Meta-analysis of continuous outcomes combining individual patient data and aggregate data. Stat Med, 2008, 27(11): 1870-1893.

69. Riley RD, Steyerberg EW. Meta-analysis of a binary outcome using individual participant data and aggregate data. Res Synth Methods, 2010, 1(1): 2-19.

70. Light RJ, Pillemer DB. Summing up: The science of reviewing research. 1984, Cambridge, MA: Harvard University Press.

71. Greenland S, Lanes S, Jara M. Estimating effects from randomized trials with discontinuations: the need for intent-to-treat design and G-estimation. Clin Trials, 2008, 5(1): 5-13.

72. Toh S, Hernan MA. Causal inference from longitudinal studies with baseline randomization. Int J Biostat, 2008, 4(1): Article 22.

73. Toh S, Hernandez-Diaz S, Logan R, Robins JM, Hernan MA. Estimating absolute risks in the presence of nonadherence: an application to a follow-up study with baseline randomization. Epidemiology, 2010, 21(4): 528-539.

74. Hernan MA, Hernandez-Diaz S. Beyond the intention-to-treat in comparative effectiveness research. Clin Trials, 2012, 9(1): 48-55.

75. Montedori A, Bonacini MI, Casazza G, Luchetta ML, Duca P, Cozzolino F, Abraha I. Modified versus standard intention-to-treat reporting: are there differences in methodological quality, sponsorship, and findings in randomized trials? A cross-sectional study. Trials, 2011, 12: 58.

76. Lewis JA, Machin D. Intention to treat–who should use ITT? Br J Cancer, 1993, 68(4): 647-650.

77. Cooper AJ, Lettis S, Chapman CL, Evans SJ, Waller PC, Shakir S, Payvandi N, Murray AB. Developing tools for the safety specification in risk management plans: lessons learned from a pilot project. Pharmacoepidemiol Drug Saf, 2008, 17(5): 445-454.

78. O'Neill RT. Assessment of safety. in Biopharmaceutical Statistics for Drug Development. 1988, Marcel Dekker.

79. Proschan MA, Lan KK, Wittes JT. Statistical Methods for Monitoring Clinical Trials. 2006, New York: Springer.

80. MedDRA Home Page. Medical Dictionary for Regulatory Activities. MedDRA MSSO (Medical Dictionary for Regulatory Activities Maintenance and Support Services Organization), 2015, 2013. http://www.meddra.org/.

81. U.S. Food and Drug Administration. Guidance for Industry: Suicidal Ideation and Behavior: Prospective Assessment of Occurrence in Clinical Trials, August 2012, accessed at. 2012. http://www.fda.gov/drugs/guidancecomplianceregulatoryinformation/guidances/ucm315156.htm.

82. Posner K, Oquendo MA, Gould M, Stanley B, Davies M. Columbia Classification Algorithm of Suicide Assessment (C-CASA): classification of suicidal events in the FDA's pediatric suicidal risk analysis of antidepressants. Am J Psychiatry, 2007, 164(7): 1035-1043.

83. Golder S, McIntosh HM, Loke Y. Identifying systematic reviews of the adverse effects of health care interventions. BMC Med Res Methodol, 2006, 6: 22.

84. Sherman RB, Woodcock J, Norden J, Grandinetti C, Temple RJ. New FDA regulation to improve safety reporting in clinical trials. N Engl J Med, 2011, 365(1): 3-5.

85. ICH International Conference on Harmonisation. ICH E3 Guideline: Structure and Content of Clinical Study Reports. 1995. http://www.ich.org/fileadmin/Public_Web_Site/ICH_Products/Guidelines/Efficacy/E3/E3_Guideline.pdf.

86. Huang HY, Andrews E, Jones J, Skovron ML, Tilson H. Pitfalls in meta-analyses on adverse events reported from clinical trials. Pharmacoepidemiol Drug Saf, 2011, 20(10): 1014-1020.

87. Loke YK, Price D, Herxheimer A, Group CAEM. Systematic reviews of adverse effects: framework for a structured approach. BMC Med Res Methodol, 2007, 7: 32.

88. ICH International Conference on Harmonisation. ICH M4E Guideline on Enhancing the Format and Structure of Benefit-Risk Information in ICH. 2014. http://www.ich.org/products/ctd/ctdsingle/article/revision-of-m4e-guideline-on-enhancing-the-format-and-structure-of-benefit-risk-information-in-ich.html.

89. U.S. Food and Drug Administration. Guidance for Industry: Premarketing Risk Assessment. 2012. http://www.fda.gov/downloads/RegulatoryInformation/Guidances/UCM126958.pdf.

90. Egger M, Zellweger-Zahner T, Schneider M, Junker C, Lengeler C, Antes G. Language bias in randomised controlled trials published in English and German. Lancet, 1997, 350(9074): 326-329.

91. Institute of Medicine. Finding What Works in Health Care: Standards for Systematic Reviews. 2011, Washington, DC: The National Academies Press.

92. Jones AP, Remmington T, Williamson PR, Ashby D, Smyth RL. High prevalence but low impact of data extraction and reporting errors were found in Cochrane systematic reviews. J Clin Epidemiol, 2005, 58(7): 741-742.

93. Horton J, Vandermeer B, Hartling L, Tjosvold L, Klassen TP, Buscemi N. Systematic review data extraction: cross-sectional study showed that experience did not increase accuracy. J Clin Epidemiol, 2010, 63(3): 289-298.

94. Buscemi N, Hartling L, Vandermeer B, Tjosvold L, Klassen TP. Single data extraction generated more errors than double data extraction in systematic reviews. J Clin Epidemiol, 2006, 59(7): 697-703.

95. Centre for Reviews and Dissemination. Systematic reviews: CRD's guidance for undertaking reviews in health care. 2009. www.york.ac.uk/media/crd/Systematic_Reviews.pdf.

96. Ware JH, Vetrovec GW, Miller AB, Van Tosh A, Gaffney M, Yunis C, Arteaga C, Borer JS. Cardiovascular safety of varenicline: patient-level meta-analysis of randomized, blinded, placebo-controlled trials. Am J Ther, 2013, 20(3): 235-246.

97. Shuster JJ. Empirical vs natural weighting in random effects meta-analysis. Stat Med, 2010, 29(12): 1259-1265.

98. Berlin JA, Kim C. The use of meta-analysis in pharmacoepidemiology. in Pharmacoepidemiology, Fourth, S.B. (ed), Editor. 2005, John Wiley and Sons: Chichester. 681-707.

99. Colditz GA, Berkey CS, Mosteller F, Brewer TF, Wilson ME, Burdick E, Fineberg HV. The efficacy of bacillus Calmette-Guerin vaccination of newborns and infants in the prevention of tuberculosis: meta-analyses of the published literature. Pediatrics, 1995, 96(1 Pt 1): 29-35.

100. Colditz GA, Brewer TF, Berkey CS, Wilson ME, Burdick E, Fineberg HV, Mosteller F. Efficacy of BCG vaccine in the prevention of tuberculosis. Meta-analysis of the published literature. JAMA, 1994, 271(9): 698-702.

101. Furukawa TA, Streiner DL, Hori S. Discrepancies among megatrials. J Clin Epidemiol, 2000, 53(12): 1193-1199.

102. LeLorier J, Grégoire G, Benhaddad A, Lapierre J, Derderian F. Discrepancies between meta-analyses and subsequent large randomized, controlled trials. N Engl J Med, 1997, 337(8): 536-542.

103. U.S. Food and Drug Administration. Statistical review and evaluation antiepileptic drugs and suicidality. 2008, 45. http://www.fda.gov/Drugs/DrugSafety/PostmarketDrugSafetyInformationforPatientsandProviders/DrugSafetyInformationforHeathcareProfessionals/ucm070651.htm.

104. Senn SJ. Overstating the evidence: double counting in meta-analysis and related problems. BMC Med Res Methodol, 2009, 9(10).

105. Thompson SG, Higgins JP. How should meta-regression analyses be undertaken and interpreted? Stat Med, 2002, 21(11): 1559-1573.

106. Gleser LJ, Olkin I. Stochastically dependent effect sizes. in The handbook of research synthesis and meta-analysis, 2nd, H. Cooper, L.V. Hedges, and J.C. Valentine, Editors. 1994, Russell Sage Foundation: New York.

107. Berlin JA, Colditz GA. The role of meta-analysis in the regulatory process for foods, drugs, and devices. JAMA, 1999, 281(9): 830-834.

108. Temple R. Meta-analysis and epidemiologic studies in drug development and postmarketing surveillance. JAMA, 1999, 281(9): 841-844.
109. Hernandez AV, Walker E, Ioannidis JP, Kattan MW. Challenges in meta-analysis of randomized clinical trials for rare harmful cardiovascular events: the case of rosiglitazone. Am Heart J, 2008, 156(1): 23-30.
110. Feinstein AR. Meta-analysis: statistical alchemy for the 21st century. J Clin Epidemiol, 1995, 48(1): 71-79.
111. Chalmers TC. Problems induced by meta-analyses. Stat Med, 1991, 10(6): 971-979; discussion 979-980.
112. Moher D, Jadad AR, Nichol G, Penman M, Tugwell P, Walsh S. Assessing the quality of randomized controlled trials: an annotated bibliography of scales and checklists. Control Clin Trials, 1995, 16(1): 62-73.
113. Chalmers TC, Smith H, Blackburn B, Silverman B, Schroeder B, Reitman D, Ambroz A. A method for assessing the quality of a randomized control trial. Control Clin Trials, 1981, 2(1): 31-49.
114. Olivo SA, Macedo LG, Gadotti IC, Fuentes J, Stanton T, Magee DJ. Scales to assess the quality of randomized controlled trials: a systematic review. Phys Ther, 2008, 88(2): 156-175.
115. Juni P, Altman DG, Egger M. Systematic reviews in health care: Assessing the quality of controlled clinical trials. BMJ, 2001, 323(7303): 42-46.
116. Borghouts JA, Koes BW, Bouter LM. The clinical course and prognostic factors of non-specific neck pain: a systematic review. Pain, 1998, 77(1): 1-13.
117. Greenland S. Quality scores are useless and potentially misleading: reply to "Re: A critical look at some popular analytic methods". Am J Epidemiol, 1994, 140(3): 300-301.
118. Fabricatore AN, Wadden TA, Moore RH, Butryn ML, Gravallese EA, Erondu NE, Heymsfield SB, Nguyen AM. Attrition from randomized controlled trials of pharmacological weight loss agents: a systematic review and analysis. Obes Rev, 2009, 10(3): 333-341.
119. Rosenbaum PR, Rubin DB. Assessing sensitivity to an unobserved binary covariate in an observational study with binary outcome. J R Stat Soc, 1983: 212-218.
120. Lin DY, Psaty BM, Kronmal RA. Assessing the sensitivity of regression results to unmeasured confounders in observational studies. Biometrics, 1998, 54(3): 948-963.
121. Schneeweiss S, Glynn RJ, Tsai EH, Avorn J, Solomon DH. Adjusting for unmeasured confounders in pharmacoepidemiologic claims data using external information: the example of COX2 inhibitors and myocardial infarction. Epidemiology, 2005, 16(1): 17-24.
122. Sturmer T, Schneeweiss S, Avorn J, Glynn RJ. Adjusting effect estimates for unmeasured confounding with validation data using propensity score calibration. Am J Epidemiol, 2005, 162(3): 279-289.
123. Kesten S, Plautz M, Piquette CA, Habib MP, Niewoehner DE. Premature discontinuation of patients: a potential bias in COPD clinical trials. Eur Respir J, 2007, 30(5): 898-906.
124. Montgomery SA, Baldwin DS, Riley A. Antidepressant medications: a review of the evidence for drug-induced sexual dysfunction. J Affect Disord, 2002, 69(1-3): 119-140.
125. Garbe E, Suissa S. Hormone replacement therapy and acute coronary outcomes: methodological issues between randomized and observational studies. Hum Reprod, 2004, 19(1): 8-13.
126. Ioannidis JP, Lau J. Completeness of safety reporting in randomized trials: an evaluation of 7 medical areas. JAMA, 2001, 285(4): 437-443.
127. Pitrou I, Boutron I, Ahmad N, Ravaud P. Reporting of safety results in published reports of randomized controlled trials. Arch Intern Med, 2009, 169(19): 1756-1761.
128. Michele TM, Pinheiro S, Iyasu S. The safety of tiotropium–the FDA's conclusions. N Engl J Med, 2010, 363(12): 1097-1099.
129. Mallinckrodt C, Chuang-Stein C, McSorley P, Schwartz J, Archibald DG, Perahia DG, Detke MJ, Alphs L. A case study comparing a randomized withdrawal trial and a double-blind long-term trial for assessing the long-term efficacy of an antidepressant. Pharm Stat, 2007, 6(1): 9-22.
130. Perahia DG, Maina G, Thase ME, Spann ME, Wang F, Walker DJ, Detke MJ. Duloxetine in the prevention of depressive recurrences: a randomized, double-blind, placebo-controlled trial. J Clin Psychiatry, 2009, 70(5): 706-716.
131. Ghaemi SN. The failure to know what isn't known: negative publication bias with lamotrigine and a glimpse inside peer review. Evid Based Ment Health, 2009, 12(3): 65-68.
132. Egger M, Davey Smith G, Schneider M, Minder C. Bias in meta-analysis detected by a simple, graphical test. BMJ, 1997, 315(7109): 629-634.
133. Sterne JA, Harbord RM. Funnel plots in meta-analysis. Stata Journal, 2004, 4: 127-141.
134. U.S. National Institutes for Health. ClinicalTrials.gov. 2007, ClinicalTrials.gov is a registry and results database of publicly and privately supported clinical studies of human participants conducted around the world. https://clinicaltrials.gov/.
135. Yahav D, Paul M, Fraser A, Sarid N, Leibovici L. Efficacy and safety of cefepime: a systematic review and meta-analysis. Lancet Infect Dis, 2007, 7(5): 338-348.
136. Brocklebank D, Wright J, Cates C. Systematic review of clinical effectiveness of pressurised metered dose inhalers versus other hand held inhaler devices for delivering corticosteroids in asthma. BMJ, 2001, 323(7318): 896-900.

137. Olkin I, Sampson A. Comparison of meta-analysis versus analysis of variance of individual patient data. Biometrics, 1998, 54(1): 317-322.

138. Szczech LA, Berlin JA, Feldman HI. The effect of antilymphocyte induction therapy on renal allograft survival. A meta-analysis of individual patient-level data. Anti-Lymphocyte Antibody Induction Therapy Study Group. Ann Intern Med, 1998, 128(10): 817-826.

139. Berlin JA, Santanna J, Schmid CH, Szczech LA, Feldman HI, Anti-Lymphocyte Antibody Induction Therapy Study G. Individual patient- versus group-level data meta-regressions for the investigation of treatment effect modifiers: ecological bias rears its ugly head. Stat Med, 2002, 21(3): 371-387.

140. Lambert PC, Sutton AJ, Abrams KR, Jones DR. A comparison of summary patient-level covariates in meta-regression with individual patient data meta-analysis. J Clin Epidemiol, 2002, 55(1): 86-94.

141. Schmid CH, Stark PC, Berlin JA, Landais P, Lau J. Meta-regression detected associations between heterogeneous treatment effects and study-level, but not patient-level, factors. J Clin Epidemiol, 2004, 57(7): 683-697.

142. Vandenbroucke JP. What is the best evidence for determining harms of medical treatment? CMAJ, 2006, 174(5): 645-646.

143. Gagne JJ, Schneeweiss S. Comment on ,empirical assessment of methods for risk identification in healthcare data: results from the experiments of the Observational Medical Outcomes Partnership'. Stat Med, 2013, 32(6): 1073-1074.

144. Rothman K, Greenland S, Lash T. Modern Epidemiology. 3rd Edition ed. 2008, Philadelphia, PA: Lippincott, Williams & Wilkins.

145. Strom BL. Study Designs Available for Pharmacoepidemiology Studies. in Pharmacoepidemiology, Fourth (4th). 2006, John Wiley & Sons.

146. Pearce N. Classification of epidemiological study designs. Int J Epidemiol, 2012, 41(2): 393-7.

147. Loke YK, Golder SP, Vandenbroucke JP. Comprehensive evaluations of the adverse effects of drugs: importance of appropriate study selection and data sources. Ther Adv Drug Saf, 2011, 2(2): 59-68.

148. Golder S, Loke YK, Bland M. Meta-analyses of adverse effects data derived from randomised controlled trials as compared to observational studies: methodological overview. PLoS Med, 2011, 8(5): e1001026.

149. Papanikolaou PN, Christidi GD, Ioannidis JP. Comparison of evidence on harms of medical interventions in randomized and nonrandomized studies. CMAJ, 2006, 174(5): 635-641.

150. Neyarapally GA, Hammad TA, Pinheiro SP, Iyasu S. Review of quality assessment tools for the evaluation of pharmacoepidemiological safety studies. BMJ open, 2012, 2(5).

151. ENCePP. European Network of Centres for Pharmacoepidemiology and Pharmacovigilance. 2006. http://www.encepp.eu/encepp/studiesDatabase.jsp.

152. Chavers S, Fife D, Wacholtz M, Stang P, Berlin J. Registration of Observational Studies: perspectives from an industry-based epidemiology group. Pharmacoepidemiol Drug Saf, 2011, 20(10): 1009-1013.

153. von Elm E, Altman DG, Egger M, Pocock SJ, Gøtzsche PC, Vandenbroucke JP, Initiative S. The Strengthening the Reporting of Observational Studies in Epidemiology (STROBE) statement: guidelines for reporting observational studies. Epidemiology, 2007, 18(6): 800-804.

154. Collaborative Group on Hormonal Factors in Breast Cancer. Breast cancer and hormone replacement therapy: collaborative reanalysis of data from 51 epidemiological studies of 52,705 women with breast cancer and 108,411 women without breast cancer. Collaborative Group on Hormonal Factors in Breast Cancer. Lancet, 1997, 350(9084): 1047-1059.

155. Salanti G, Dias S, Welton NJ, Ades AE, Golfinopoulos V, Kyrgiou M, Mauri D, Ioannidis JP. Evaluating novel agent effects in multiple-treatments meta-regression. Stat Med, 2010, 29(23): 2369-2383.

156. Bucher HC, Guyatt GH, Griffith LE, Walter SD. The results of direct and indirect treatment comparisons in meta-analysis of randomized controlled trials. J Clin Epidemiol, 1997, 50(6): 683-691.

157. Lumley T. Network meta-analysis for indirect treatment comparisons. Stat Med, 2002, 21(16): 2313-2324.

158. Lu G, Ades A. Assessing evidence inconsistency in mixed treatment comparisons. Journal of the American Statistical Association, 2006, 101(474).

159. Higgins JP, Jackson D, Barrett JK, Lu G, Ades AE, White IR. Consistency and inconsistency in network meta-analysis: concepts and models for multi-arm studies. Res Synth Methods, 2012, 3(2): 98-110.

160. Donegan S, Williamson P, D'Alessandro U, Tudur Smith C. Assessing key assumptions of network meta-analysis: a review of methods. Res Synth Methods, 2013, 4(4): 291-323.

161. Coxib and traditional NSAID Trialists' (CNT) Collaboration, Bhala N, Emberson J, Merhi A, Abramson S, Arber N, Baron JA, et al. Vascular and upper gastrointestinal effects of non-steroidal anti-inflammatory drugs: meta-analyses of individual participant data from randomised trials. Lancet, 2013, 382(9894): 769-779.

162. Mills EJ, Thorlund K, Ioannidis JP. Demystifying trial networks and network meta-analysis. BMJ, 2013, 346: f2914.

CHAPTER 4.

ANALYSIS AND REPORTING

This chapter is intended to provide guidance on the analysis and reporting associated with meta-analyses of safety data as well as information on the technical aspects of data analysis. Extensive examination of these technical aspects is not in the scope of this chapter as in-depth details are available elsewhere for those who may be interested. However, practical implications and importance of the analytical choices are described. This chapter is rather technical, although interpretive context is provided.

Some of the major areas covered in this chapter are issues related to measures of treatment effect, challenges in dealing with rare events, considerations for the choice of the appropriate statistical model, advantages and disadvantage of Bayesian approaches, issues around power calculations and missing data, considerations regarding multiplicity, heterogeneity, meta-regression and sensitivity analyses. Finally, the chapter provides a proposed checklist for reporting of meta-analysis of drug safety.

4.1 Measures of treatment effect

Summary of main points:

▶ The outcome measure chosen may influence the statistical significance or the level of uncertainty of the primary result or may affect the apparent degree of statistical heterogeneity.

▶ Various effect estimates describing efficacy and safety are available, depending on the specific type of data.

▶ In choosing a scale for an overall treatment effect, it is important to consider the consistency of effect across studies, mathematical properties and ease of interpretation. Absolute measures (e.g. risk differences) capture the public health implications of interventions better than relative measures. On the other hand, relative measures also have advantages. For example, empirical studies have demonstrated less statistical heterogeneity of the relative measures than the risk difference measures between studies in the same meta-analysis. It will often be helpful to express estimated effects on both absolute and relative scales.

Depending on the specific type of data, various effect estimates (whether describing efficacy or safety) are available. The point estimates and CIs for these effects comprise the backbone for a typical meta-analysis. The following paragraphs discuss consistency of effect across studies, mathematical properties and ease of interpretation of potential metrics (as recommended by Deeks & Altman [163] and Sutton et al. [164]) for several kinds of data.

Continuous data. Quantitative measures, typically summarized using means and standard deviations, are often the primary and/or secondary outcomes of interest for a clinical trial to treat a metabolic disease, such as blood pressure for a hypertension trial or percentage of HbA1c in total haemoglobin for a diabetes trial. Under these scenarios, efficacy for a particular dose of active drug treatment is often defined as the difference in the change (or percentage change) from baseline in the outcome, at a specified point in time, between an experimental treatment and a control group (either placebo or standard of care). Continuous variables may also be indicators of safety (e.g. blood pressure might be increased by a drug that is indicated for sinus congestion). Continuous data are among the easiest to analyse as many statistical methods can be used. As they can often be summarized with well-known statistics such as the sample mean or sample mean difference, they are typically easy to interpret.

Binary data. Binary outcomes are classified into two categories (e.g. yes vs. no, or response vs. non-response). Results are typically summarized as proportions (the number with the event divided by the number of participants at risk for the event), while measures of treatment effect are typically given as a risk difference (the difference between two proportions), risk ratio (the ratio of one proportion to another) or odds ratio (the ratio of one "odds" divided by another, where the "odds" of an event is a proportion divided by one minus the proportion). The risk difference (RD) is an absolute measure, while the risk ratio (RR) and odds ratio (OR) are relative measures. (We use the term "relative risk" in this report to represent a more general concept that could include RR, odds ratio, hazard ratio, rate ratio, etc.). Definitions are given in the Glossary (Annex I). One would typically work with the event proportions from each intervention group within each study. However, statistical methods are also available to enable working directly with the treatment effect measures (e.g. OR, RR or RD). Such direct use of these measures also requires estimates of their variability (CIs or standard errors) within each study.

For rare events, the RR and OR will be very close to each other numerically. When there are no events in either arm of a study, a relative outcome measure provides no information about the relative event rates, although Bayesian methods make some use of these data. Meta-analyses using RR or OR as the effect measure traditionally include studies with zero events in either arm, but not both. Studies with zero events in both arms do not provide information regarding RR or OR and often mathematically are dropped from the meta-analysis. Thus, summaries of RDs may, in some circumstances, be based on more studies than summaries of relative risks because they include studies with zero events in either or both arms.

Empirical studies have demonstrated less statistical heterogeneity of the relative measures than the RD measures between studies in the same meta-analysis [165, 166] – i.e. relative measures tend to be less variable across studies than are RDs. However, the RDs are generally viewed as more clinically interpretable. They reflect the public health impact better than relative measures as they lead to calculations of excess numbers of events. Depending on the availability of IPD and the willingness to assume constancy of the effect size across trials, one might conduct the analysis using more than one metric (e.g. ORs and RDs), or conduct the analysis on one scale (e.g. OR) and then convert the summary measure to another metric. Localio et al. propose a method for converting from OR to other metrics [167]. This kind of approach could be useful in helping understand the public health and benefit–risk implications of the results of the meta-analysis. The interpretation of an RD of 2% would be different if it represents 3% minus 1% vs. 60% minus 58% and hence is tied with baseline risk. Similarly, a relative risk of 3 could be observed when the event rate in exposed patients is 3 per 10 000 compared with 1 per 10 000 in unexposed patients, or when the exposed risk is 30% compared with 10% in unexposed patients. These two situations have very different implications (see section 5.5.1).

It should be noted that the results remain invariant under switching the coding of the event and non-event for OR and RD but not for RR. That is, switching the coding of the event and non-event can make a substantial difference for RRs, affecting the effect size, its significance and observed heterogeneity. (See Deeks [165] for a discussion of when to select the event vs. non-event.) This is not the case for RD (for which a coding switch changes only the sign of the effect) or OR (for which a coding switch yields an effect that is the reciprocal of the original OR).

Rates. Count data are sometimes summarized as incidence rates (events per person-time). In this case, measures of treatment effect will typically be either a rate difference or a rate ratio, in an analogous manner to RD and RR above.

Number needed to treat for benefit and number needed to treat for harm. Although not commonly used in meta-analysis, the number needed to treat (NNT) for benefit is another way of expressing the benefit of a new treatment in binary response data over a given time period. It is simply the reciprocal of the difference between two proportions (i.e. the proportions of the outcome in question in each of two treatment groups). In a clinical trial setting, it can be interpreted as the number of patients who need to be treated, on average, in order to prevent/promote one additional outcome over a given time period. The number needed to treat for harm is a similar concept, but is the NNT, on average, to induce one additional AE over a given time period. Even when not part of a meta-analysis, there are statistical challenges with using NNT [168], particularly with respect to calculation of CIs. Thus it is not recommended to combine studies using NNT directly. Another idea would be to take a single pooled RD from a meta-analysis and calculate an NNT from it. However, such a pooled NNT may not be very useful to clinicians because the "true" NNT might vary substantially in differing patient subgroups. In cases where the relative risk reduction is reasonably constant across trials in the meta-analysis (or subgroups of trials), applying the pooled relative risk reductions (calculated from all trials in the meta-analysis or from subgroups of trials) to the baseline risk relevant to specific patient groups, in order to calculate a range of NNTs can be useful and informative. See Smeeth et al. for examples of this calculation [169].

Time-to-event data. The hazard ratio usually serves as the primary effect measure for group comparisons with time-to-event data. Hazard ratios are not always reported, so that meta-analysis of time-to-event data can be challenging when relying on published data from published results. Calculating hazard ratios may therefore sometimes depend on the availability of individual subject-level data. A variety of transformations and approximations have been proposed for dealing with other summary statistics that are often reported in published studies [170] and for extracting information from survival curves [171, 172]. The digitized survival curves can also be utilized to extract data from published papers. Also, when the hazard ratio is not reported for some studies, there can be a temptation to treat the endpoint as binary. Note that the choice of metric can have an impact on how the trial is weighted. When the event rate is high the precision of the hazard ratio estimate is high, but the precision of the OR estimate is low. Using the OR can underweight the study substantially compared with the hazard ratio (if the meta-analysis is using a method that weights studies according to the inverse of variance).

Ordinal outcome data. Although ordinal outcome data are occasionally seen in clinical studies of neuroscience therapies, such as a patient self-reported ordinal score reflecting the degree of the headache he/she is suffering from, meta-analysis of ordinal data is less common than meta-analysis of binary or continuous data [173] and it is rare to have access to the required data [174].

The above discussed outcome measures can be used for both summary-level and IPD meta-analysis, but clearly there is more flexibility when IPD are available. Also, a continuous variable may be dichotomized and analysed as a binary outcome (or rate). For example, in a study of a cholesterol-lowering drug, the LDL-C measurement at the study end can be dichotomized into "yes" or "no" depending on whether it is below a certain target level (such as 100 mg/dL) or not. Survival data (i.e. data where the outcome variable is the time until the occurrence of an event of interest) may be analysed as time-to-event or as an OR, if the duration of all studies is similar. The nature of the outcome and biological mechanism may influence the choice between RR, rate ratio and hazard ratio. For summary-level meta-analysis, where effect estimates are available for each individual study based on the analyses conducted by the original authors, a challenge is that there can be several effect measures to choose from and different ways of estimating each. With access to the IPD, the analyst generally has a great deal of flexibility to estimate effect sizes using whatever metric is most appropriate to answer the clinical questions being asked. Section 9.4.4.4 of the Cochrane Handbook gives general advice regarding points to consider when choosing a measure for binary outcomes.

For participant-level meta-analysis, in which the same outcome measures are collected consistently for each participant across all included studies, the choice of an effect measure would still require considerations such as clinical interpretability of the effect measure. In addition to clinical considerations, there are also statistical considerations. The outcome measure chosen may influence the statistical significance of the primary result or may affect the apparent degree of heterogeneity. This emphasizes the need for planning based on statistical and clinical principles. There should be a planned primary approach along with sensitivity analyses to assess the robustness of conclusions reached.

For some types of outcome measures (e.g. patient-reported outcomes), there may be multiple assessment tools (scales) available. In such circumstances, a standardized mean difference, expressed in standard deviation units (the so-called "effect size"), may be needed. Methods for working with these standardized mean differences can be found in Hedges & Olkin [175].

4.2 Statistical methods for rare-event meta-analysis

Summary of main points:

▶ Low event counts pose unique statistical challenges. These include:

— When one or both arms of a study have zero events, relative metrics (such as the log OR and log RR) become undefined within-study, as do their variances. This makes combining information from those studies with the other studies challenging.

— Standard inferences for meta-analysis rely on large sample approximations. They may not be valid statistically when the total number of AEs is low or the number of AEs in any single study is low.

▶ The choice of method in a low-event meta-analysis is important since certain methods perform poorly with respect to bias and CI coverage:

— Inverse variance and DerSimonian and Laird methods are not generally recommended for the analysis of rare events.

— Continuity corrections can help with the problem of zero events in a single arm, but the standard correction of adding a constant (usually 0.5) to all cells of the 2x2 table is the least desirable correction [176, 177].

— Bayesian methods show promise for analysing rare event analysis.

▶ If one uses off-the-shelf software to do a meta-analysis of low-frequency events, it is particularly important to understand what the software is actually doing. Many software packages have automatic handling of zero cells. If the software offers only automatic handling of zero cells using suboptimal methods, it may be wise to consider alternative software.

Evaluations of rare events that result in important health consequences are common in safety assessment. Meta-analysis of data on rare AEs presents some unique statistical challenges. In this section we discuss some of the challenges, caveats and potential solutions for analysis of AEs with low frequency.

Standard inferences for meta-analysis rely on large sample approximations. They may not be valid statistically when the total number of events is low or the number of events in any single study is low. If the number of studies included in the meta-analysis is small or modest, the statistical test for heterogeneity generally has low power.

When one or both arms of a study have zero events, the log OR and log RR become undefined, as do their variances and this causes problems with several potential analysis methods. To overcome this problem, a continuity correction factor is often added to each cell of the 2×2 table for the studies with zero events in either arm. However there is no consensus regarding how to handle double-zero (or even single-zero) studies when the analysis metric is relative (e.g. RR, OR or hazard ratio). When there are no events in either arm of a study, a relative outcome measure provides no information about the relative event rates. The next few paragraphs outline some of the differing techniques and perspectives.

Various statistical methods for rare-event meta-analysis are addressed in a few recent papers [176-181]. Sutton et al. discussed several important issues as they relate to model choice, continuity corrections, exact statistics, Bayesian methods and sensitivity analysis [164].

Some of the many publications that address rare events in meta-analysis are described below.

Sweeting et al. [176, 177] compared the performance of different meta-analysis methods for combining ORs with an emphasis on the use of continuity corrections. They dropped the double-zero studies and added continuity correction to single-zero studies only. They noted that "[a] preliminary investigation that preceded the main simulation study described here, by analysing data sets both including and excluding such studies using the Bayesian model that does not require continuity correction factors, confirmed that zero total event studies do not contribute to a fixed-effect meta-analysis". They studied constant correction factors as well as two alternative continuity corrections. They found that the standard continuity correction factor of adding a fixed value of 0.5 to each cell of the 2x2 table that is used routinely (and implemented in most software) may not perform well, especially when the treatment groups are of substantially different sizes (i.e. the randomization ratio is much different from 1:1). They concluded that the two alternative continuity corrections outperformed the constant correction factor in nearly all situations. They also found that the inverse variance method performed consistently poorly, irrespective of the continuity correction used.

Bradburn et al. [179] evaluated the performance of 10 meta-analysis methods (seven for combining ORs and three for combining RDs) with rare events for binary outcomes. They also excluded double-zero studies for ORs because the trial "provides no information about either the likely direction or magnitude of the effect". They suggested that the choice of statistical method depends on the underlying event rate, the likely size of the treatment effect and consideration of balance in the numbers of treated and control participants in the studies. They found that the bias was greatest in inverse-variance, the DerSimonian and Laird method, and the Mantel-Haenszel OR method using a 0.5 constant continuity correction. At event rates below 1% (for the sample sizes studied), the Peto OR method [182] provided the least biased, most powerful estimate and best CI coverage provided there was no substantial imbalance between treatment and control group sizes within studies, and treatment effects were not exceptionally large. Bradburn et al. noted that Greenland & Salvan [183] demonstrated considerable bias with the Peto method with imbalances between the numbers in the two groups of 8:1 or greater and ORs of above 2.5, and in a randomized matched-pair trial with ORs of around 5. However, such scenarios are rarely encountered in the meta-analysis of RCTs. In other circumstances, the Mantel-Haenszel OR method without zero-cell correction, logistic regression and the exact stratified OR method generally performed well and were less biased than the Peto method. They found that the Mantel-Haenszel RD method produced relatively unbiased estimates of treatment effects. However, all the RD methods yielded CIs that were too wide (and had associated poor statistical power) when events were rare. The coverage of the CIs degenerated to 100% coverage at the lowest event rates.

Tian et al. [180] proposed an exact inference fixed-effect procedure for calculating RDs that includes zero-event studies. Cai et al. [184] proposed an unconditional approach (by including zero-event studies) based on the Poisson random-effects model in the rare event setting. Bennett et al. [178] compared Bayesian and frequentist meta-analytical approaches for analysing time to event data. They studied three main methods. The first was the standard Cox Proportional hazards method. The second was a penalized Cox Proportional Hazards method (Heinze & Schemper method with Firth correction), which was first used by Firth (1993) [185] and then applied to the Cox model by Heinze & Schemper [186]. The third was a Bayesian proportional hazards method (with diffuse prior and informative prior). They found that the Firth correction method outperformed the other methods studied.

Bayesian methods can be appropriately applied to rare events meta-analysis. The use of hierarchical models can modulate the extremes in the zero event setting, borrowing information from studies with events to derive posterior inferences for the treatment effect estimates. A practical challenge of Bayesian meta-analysis for rare AE data is that non-informative priors may lead to convergence failure due to very sparse data. Weakly informative priors, which put weak restrictions on the size of the treatment effect, may be used to solve this issue. For example, assuming a prior distribution for no treatment effect with a mean log (RR) of 0 and a standard deviation of 2, this roughly translates to an assumption that we are 95% sure that the RR for treatment effect is between 0.02 and 55, with an estimate of the mean RR of 1.0. Although this prior is not non-informative, it is reasonably weak in the sense that it specifies a wide range of possible values for RR from 0.02 to 55. To further consider some sceptical priors that are arguably more sensible in the safety setting, we can assume an effect of two-fold risk (i.e. $\log(RR) = 0.7$) with two different standard deviations of 2 or 0.7. These two priors translate into a 95% CI for the RR of (0.04, 110) and (0.5, 8.2), respectively. By using these three weakly informative priors as sensitivity analyses, we can assess the robustness of the results against different choices of priors.

Sensitivity analysis (see section 4.9 for more details of sensitivity analyses) is especially important in the rare AE setting, because results may be sensitive to both statistical and non-statistical considerations. With respect to statistical issues, choice of statistical methods, scale of measurement, prior specification if the Bayesian approach is utilized, and continuity correction factors selected for analysing zero-events studies should all be evaluated.

If one is using off-the-shelf software to do a meta-analysis of low-frequency events, it is particularly important to understand what the software is actually doing. Many software packages have automatic handling of zero cells and there is no opportunity to utilize, for instance, the alternate continuity corrections that were found by Sweeting et al. [176, 177] to offer better statistical properties. If the software offers only automatic handling of zero cells using suboptimal methods, it may be wise to consider alternative software.

4.3   Choice of statistical model

Summary of main points:

▶ Fixed-effect and random-effects models address different research questions. The choice of model is determined by whether the variability within study alone or the variability both within and between studies is required to answer the research question.

▶ Random-effects models yield a more uniform weighting of the individual study estimates than will a fixed-effect model.

▶ The decision to use a fixed-effect or random-effects model should be specified in the meta-analysis protocol. Regardless of the primary model, the reasons for any heterogeneity of the treatment effect across studies should be explored.

▶ The choice of fixed-effect or random-effects model should not depend on heterogeneity. The degree of heterogeneity of treatment effects between studies is an important result in a meta-analysis and should be interpreted in the clinical context.

▶ In a random-effects model the method of estimating the between-study variance is important. The method of DerSimonian and Laird, or the inclusion of the study-specific treatment effects as a random effect in a general mixed-effects model, are two of the possibilities, at least when the data are not sparse.

The choice of statistical model and more generally the choice of statistical methods in a meta-analysis may be influenced by several factors. These include the type of endpoint, availability of IPD or summary-level data, frequency of occurrence of an event, the intended populations of studies and the statistical inference to be drawn. In this section we discuss some important aspects of the choice of statistical model. This choice matters, as it can influence the point estimate of the treatment effect, as well as the width of the CI and hence the statistical significance.

4.3.1   Fixed-effect and random-effects models

Both fixed-effect and random-effects statistical methods are available for making inferences from the observed data in a meta-analysis to a larger population. The fundamental difference between them in meta-analysis concerns whether the treatment effect is included in the statistical model as a fixed effect or as a random effect. The choice of which to use, as well as the meaning of each is sometimes a contentious issue in meta-analysis [187, page 280].

The fixed-effect model is sometimes referred to (or at least is described) as a common-effects model. That is, the studies are assumed to be all estimating a single true underlying effect size. In that framework the choice between fixed effect and random effects is framed entirely as a question of heterogeneity of effect-size parameters. However, while it is true that a common effects model implies that a fixed effect model is appropriate, the converse is not true. A fixed-effect model does not imply that the studies all estimate a single true underlying effect size. There is confusion regarding this issue.

The choice of the model should be informed by the research question and the extent of the statistical inference to be drawn from the data. Each model addresses a different research question [187, page 38, 188]. If the research question is concerned with whether an estimate of the average treatment effect in the existing studies is consistent with chance or not, then only the variability within study (and hence a fixed-effect meta-analysis) is appropriate. From this perspective the fixed-effect meta-analysis is not concerned with making an inference to a hypothetical population of studies, but rather to determine the chance consequences of sampling people into the observed studies [189]. In contrast, if the research question is concerned with estimating the treatment effect from a (hypothetical) population of studies, from which the existing studies constitute an (assumed) random sample, then the variability within and among studies (and hence a random-effects meta-analysis) is required.

Viewed from the above perspective, the assumption that the studies in the meta-analysis estimate a common treatment effect is not required in a fixed-effect model. Similarly, the lack of a common treatment effect does not imply the need for a random-effects model.

In general, the random-effects model (the model that includes the study-specific treatment effects as a random effect) will result in a larger standard error for the estimate of the overall treatment effect. Viewed from the perspective of weighting the individual study results, the random-effects model will yield a more uniform weighting of the individual study estimates than will a fixed-effect model. In the presence of high heterogeneity, one should consider the appropriateness of the greater equality of weights for large and small studies as a consequence of a random-effects model, as the greater equality of weights may not be desirable. Poole & Greenland [190] present an example of a meta-analysis in which small studies and large studies give different results. They note that this situation might arise from publication bias, with small studies being published only when they show statistically significant findings (implying larger effect sizes). In such a situation, it might be inappropriate to increase the weight for the published smaller studies, as those might represent a biased subset of all small studies. It is important to stress that there is no necessary connection between weights and fixed-effect or random-effects models. The choice of weights can be informed by other considerations.

Factors to consider when defining the research question and hence the choice of a fixed-effect or random-effects model, specifically in a drug development programme, are discussed by Berlin et al. [191].

Safety meta-analyses in a regulatory setting are conducted to inform regulators of potential treatment harms for current and future patients. This often leads to the research question as to whether the estimate of harm in the existing studies is consistent with chance or not. As discussed above, this research question can be addressed by a fixed-effect meta-analysis. In a regulatory setting the choice of model should be agreed with the regulatory agencies before conducting the analysis.

Regardless of whether fixed-effect or random-effects meta-analysis is conducted, it is critical that the meta-analysis be accompanied by checks on the consistency of effects across studies (see sections 4.3.4 and 4.8). The same overall meta-analysis treatment effect estimate can arise from a set of studies with identical results as can arise from a set of studies in which the treatment effect results show that the treatment is highly harmful in some studies and is even beneficial in others. Without investigating the statistical heterogeneity of results, one could be readily misled. Peto [189] noted that

> As an example, consider the use of diethylstilbesterol (DES) as a treatment for prostate cancer. DES reduces the risk of death from prostate cancer but increases the risk of death from heart disease. Without disease-specific analyses, the hazard that this treatment confers on patients at high risk of death from myocardial infarction could easily have been missed.

A related example is in the FDA reviewer guidance [192, section 7.4.1.1] which mentions the following:

> In one case, for example, several studies were combined and a reassuringly low estimate of phototoxicity was obtained. Subsequent examination of individual study results found one study with a substantial rate of phototoxicity. The study was the only outpatient study done (i.e. the only one in which patients had an opportunity to be exposed to sunlight). In some situations, the incidence may be best described by the range in the various studies. For the phototoxicity example above, however, the most relevant data are those from the outpatient study, the only study that was conducted under conditions pertinent to intended use.

The variability of both study design and study results (heterogeneity) is discussed at greater length in section 4.8. Here we note only that a practice we have seen repeatedly in publications is to use the degree of variability as a guide to the choice of fixed-effect vs. random-effects models. That is, people sometimes use the mere presence of heterogeneity of results as a reason to use the random-effects model. We will argue, below, that this approach may not only be of questionable validity statistically, but misses the broader point that developing an understanding of sources of heterogeneity in results should become a focus of the analysis. In Appendix 2, the example of erythropoietin stimulating agents shows the investigation of heterogeneity of treatment effects.

4.3.2   Model specification/analytical methods

The analytical decision of using a fixed-effect or random-effects model should be specified in the protocol and the statistical analysis plan (SAP) for the meta-analysis. Regardless of the primary model, the reasons for any heterogeneity of the treatment effect across studies should be explored and the analytical methods for exploring heterogeneity should also be given in the SAP (see sections 4.8-4.10).

The analytical method will be influenced by the type of endpoint. In meta-analysis of treatment harm in a regulatory setting, endpoints are often binary, leading to methods appropriate for proportions, incidence rates or, if subject-level data are available, a time-to-event analysis. Less frequently, harm may be measured using continuous variables such as laboratory values. The primary outcome variable should be specified in the protocol and SAP, together with the appropriate measure of treatment effect (e.g. OR, RR, incidence rate ratio, incidence rate difference, hazard ratio or mean difference.

There are a number of appropriate methods for the analysis of summary-level binary outcome measures, both parametric (e.g. logistic regression) and non-parametric (e.g. Peto method) [182]. These methods can be utilized in either a fixed-effect or random-effects meta-analysis. Often the DerSimonian & Laird method [193] is used to estimate the between-variance of the study-specific estimates of treatment effect in the random-effects model. While this method is direct and easy to compute, it has been shown to have limitations in the case of rare events or if inferences about heterogeneity across studies are important (e.g. Jackson et al. [194]). Alternatively, general linear or non-linear mixed-effects models found in many statistical software packages (e.g. various SAS procedures) may be used to estimate the variability of treatment effect between studies. These methods usually employ likelihood or pseudo-likelihood methods to estimate the variability. Treatment effects can also be incorporated as random effects in a hierarchical Bayes model. Bayesian meta-analysis is becoming more widely used in medical research and the reader is referred to section 4.4 of this document, which discusses Bayesian methods.

More recently, an alternative method for variance estimation for random-effects models has received attention. Cornell et al. [195] provide an example in which the DerSimonian-Laird model produced a statistically significant result, whereas other models, including the so-called Knapp-Hartung model, did not yield statistical significance. Another recent publication provides a free spreadsheet that contains a simple calculation converting the results of the DerSimonian-Laird model to the Knapp-Hartung model [196]. Thus, there is potential to incorporate a fairly simple approach into more standard practice via "accessible" software.

4.3.3   Parameter estimation

This section is intended to give a brief discussion of important aspects of the estimation of the overall treatment effect in meta-analysis.

Typically in meta-analysis, each study contributes an independent estimate and corresponding variance of the outcome measure of treatment effect. In general, a weighted average of these study-specific estimates yields the overall estimate of treatment effect in the meta-analysis. As stated above, fixed-effect and random-effects models generally give rise to different study weights. For example, in a fixed-effect meta-analysis a common way of estimating the overall treatment effect is by the inverse-variance method. For this method the weights that are used to compute the weighted (meta-analysis) estimate are inversely proportional to the individual-study estimate of the variance of the treatment effect for that study.

In a random-effects model that utilizes the inverse variance method, the individual study weights are inversely proportional to the sum of the individual-study estimate of the variance of the treatment effect for that study *and* an estimate of the variance between studies. As discussed in section 4.3.2, there are various ways to estimate the between-study variance. Inspection of these two sets of weights indicates why a random-effects model can weight the individual study estimates very differently from a fixed-effect model. As noted, there can be practical implications for this choice – it is not just an academic decision. Because the choice of method can affect the statistical inference, pre-specification of the choice is essential. Sensitivity analyses and the exploration of heterogeneity of effect across studies should be conducted regardless of the choice of model.

It should be noted that the inverse-variance weights, and any set of weights, imply a relative importance to each study estimate. It may be that each of the studies included in a meta-analysis is considered to be of equal importance. In this case the SAP could specify that the studies be equally weighted. The choice of weights determines the way in which the individual study estimates are combined in order to obtain the overall estimate, while the fixed/random choice determines the appropriate variability. The weights (and more generally the analytical methods) should be consistent with the clinical question and specified beforehand in the SAP.

There are alternative methods to the methods discussed above to obtain the overall meta-estimate of treatment effect, such as Mantel-Haenszel, generalized linear and non-linear mixed models and Bayesian methods (section 4.4). If all the studies have similar estimates of the treatment effect, the fixed-effect and random-effects estimates are similar. It is only when there are considerable differences between studies in treatment effect estimates that fixed-effect and random-effects models may yield different summary estimates. Hence the general issue of heterogeneity should be explored. Funnel plots are a useful graphical tool to illustrate why the point estimates between a random-effects and fixed-effect model differ. An association between the weights employed to obtain the summary estimate and the individual treatment effects estimates can lead to different point estimates. As noted above, this can happen when small studies, which have higher weights with random-effects models, have larger effect sizes than large studies.

4.3.4 Statistical heterogeneity of treatment effects

The degree of heterogeneity of treatment effect between studies is an important result in a meta-analysis. It should be stressed that the choice of fixed-effect or random-effects model should not depend on heterogeneity or lack of heterogeneity. Nor does the use of a random-effects model obviate the need for an analysis of potential sources of heterogeneity.

A common way to test for heterogeneity is to utilize Cochran's Q Statistic [197]. Other methods, specifically for ORs, include the Breslow-Day test and Zelen's exact test for homogeneity of ORs. If model-based methods are used to estimate the treatment effect, heterogeneity may be tested via the treatment by study interaction term. Tests for heterogeneity may have low power to detect clinically-important heterogeneity when the number of studies and/or events is small or may have the power to detect clinically-meaningless heterogeneity when the number of studies or events is large [198]. This is not simply a theoretical discussion, as a regulatory action might depend on the interpretation of the degree of heterogeneity of treatment effects.

A useful descriptive measure that quantifies heterogeneity is $I^2 = 100 \frac{Q - k + 1}{Q}$, where Q is Cochran's Q statistic and is the number of studies. This statistic is interpreted as the percentage of the total variation of treatment effect between studies that is due to heterogeneity. As a relative measure, is subject to some potential idiosyncrasies. For example, in a situation when there are very large studies, the average within-study variability will likely be small, implying that even a small degree of between-study variability in effect sizes could produce a large value of . Thus, the degree of heterogeneity should be interpreted in the context of substantive clinical implications [198]. A forest plot (see section 4.10.1) can be a useful tool for visual inspection of the degree of variability between studies.

4.4 Bayesian meta-analysis

Summary of main points:

▶ Although there are many advantages of using Bayesian methods, the ability to synthesize evidence under a unified framework and to handle complex problems is one of the most important advantages of the Bayesian approach in the meta-analysis setting.

▶ While Bayesian methods are appealing, they can be computationally complex to implement. Care must be taken to check many aspects of the methodology (e.g. if Markov Chain Monte Carlo methods are used, the convergence of the Markov chain, sensitivity to specific prior distributions and initial values should all be checked) [199]. It is recommended that, whenever the Bayesian methods are employed, expertise should be sought to ensure appropriate implementation.

▶ Sensitivity analyses are particularly important for Bayesian analyses in terms of checking how influential the priors and the likelihood models are.

Bayesian statistics, originating from Bayes' theorem [200], refer to a philosophy of statistics that treats probability statements as having degrees of belief, in contrast to frequentist statistics that regard probability strictly as being based on frequencies of occurrence of events [59]. Conceptually, the Bayes' system is simple. We modify our opinions with objective information. Previous information/initial beliefs plus recent objective data yield a new and improved belief. The terminology for the parts of this equation is as follows: *prior* refers to the probability distribution of the previous information/initial beliefs; the *likelihood* function is the probability of other hypotheses with objective new data; and the *posterior* is the probability distribution of the newly revised belief [201].

There are different types of priors. For example, a prior can be "informative" to reflect someone's prior beliefs or previous (e.g. historical) data, which may be viewed as "subjective", or a prior can be "vague" or "non-informative" (e.g. when there is no relevant information available). As an example, if we were looking at a biological with immune-suppressant activity, we might have prior evidence that we would see an increase in the risk of opportunistic infections, so an informative prior can be used. In contrast, if there is no history with members of the same class of drugs for the same indication, we might need a non-informative prior.

Once a prior is specified, current data are expressed with an appropriate statistical model through the *likelihood* function. Then the *posterior probability distribution* for the quantities of interest, which can be obtained by combining the prior and the likelihood, forms the basis for the Bayesian inferences.

For both the Bayesian paradigm and meta-analysis, the goal is to incorporate all information in order to draw inference with as much accuracy as possible, to account for all the uncertainty associated with estimation, and to present the results in a manner that leads to coherent decisions.

4.4.1 Advantages and disadvantages of Bayesian methods

The Bayesian meta-analysis offers many advantages over frequentist approaches. The following bullet points summarize the main advantages and disadvantages.

Advantages of Bayesian meta-analysis

▶ Provides a unified framework for synthesizing evidence from multiple data sources/studies/treatments in a formal, consistent and coherent manner, taking all the uncertainty at different levels into account. While it is theoretically possible to do this in a frequentist framework, it is often cumbersome. Consequently, frequentist methods typically use somewhat simple models (e.g. they often assume that uncertain parameters, such as the variance of effect sizes between studies, are actually known). Markov Chain Monte Carlo (MCMC) methods in conjunction with the Bayesian hierarchical modelling approach can be used to address different, potentially complex meta-analysis problems (such as dealing with an event with non-constant hazards over time or addressing whether a risk is a class effect over several different drugs or a risk is only applicable to certain indications of a particular drug).

▶ Allows formal incorporation of other sources of evidence (such as data from historical controls or data from other drugs in the same class) by utilizing prior distributions for quantities of interest.

▶ Allows calculation of probabilities of certain hypotheses – e.g. the probability that the OR, representing a treatment effect, is less than 1.3 (for which a high probability might support the null hypothesis that the event is not caused by the drug, reminiscent of the requirement by the FDA for evaluation of cardiovascular risk in anti-diabetic drug development) [8] or at least 2 (for which a high probability might support existence of a clinically meaningful treatment effect). Calculation of probabilities such as these cannot be done in the classic frequentist framework of parameter estimation. In addition, it also provides probability statements about true treatment effects under different scales (such as OR, RR or RD) which are easier to understand than classic inferences such as P values and CIs. For example, we might be interested in the probability that an RD in mortality between drug A and drug B is greater than 1 in 1000 subjects or the probability that subjects receiving drug A have better median survival than drug B.

▶ Enables predictive statements, including an estimate of uncertainty, to be made easily.

▶ Offer additional advantages in the rare event meta-analysis setting. These are discussed in section 4.2.

Disadvantages of Bayesian meta-analysis

▶ The specification of prior distributions for the parameters of interest is one of the most difficult and controversial aspects of Bayesian meta-analysis. Critics are concerned that use of informative prior beliefs may undermine objectivity. In this context, it is important to specify informative priors carefully on the basis of objective data or to use weakly informative priors (see section 4.2). In the regulatory setting, priors based on subjective beliefs should be avoided. (However, if the priors are truly non-informative, there may be a similar frequentist analysis available, which avoids the extra work required to check that the Bayesian methods are not being influenced by the choice of prior. The exception to this is when there are complexity issues that make the Bayesian approach computationally superior, as noted in the first bullet under "Advantages").

4.4.2   Additional information

A frequentist random-effects approach to meta-analysis usually focuses on estimation of an overall treatment effect while a fully Bayesian approach estimates the overall treatment effect and also trial-specific effects (which shrink to an overall mean) and permits a variety of useful extensions. A vast literature has evolved with a particular emphasis on Bayesian random-effects models to deal with a wide variety of meta-analysis problems [199, 202-207]. All of this work focuses on dealing with different aspects of heterogeneity, either indirectly through modelling assumptions or more directly by introducing additional information together with an appropriate regression structure [208]. There are a few good practical examples of Bayesian meta-analysis. Higgins et al. [203] discuss the fact that meta-analyses of very few studies need not "default" to a fixed-effect model since informative prior distributions for the extent of heterogeneity can be incorporated in a simple Bayesian approach. Higgins & Spiegelhalter [209] applied Bayesian methods of meta-analysis to magnesium trials in myocardial infarction before and after publication of a large trial. They show how scepticism can be formally incorporated into the analysis using a prior distribution. They also showed how Bayesian meta-analysis models can be used to explore different hypotheses that treatment effect depends on the size of the trial or the underlying risk of the control group. Kalil [49] conducted a Bayesian reappraisal of the findings using the frequentist methods used by the FDA [10] and by Yahav et al. [135], showing that there is a 91% (by FDA trial-level meta-analysis), 81% (by FDA participant-level meta-analysis) and 99% (by Yahav et al. meta-analysis) probability that cefepime raises mortality in neutropenic fever patients. This example demonstrates the ability of Bayesian methods to make direct probability statements. It is also an example of how different approaches can lead to different conclusions about a safety signal. Askling et al. [210] used the Bayesian hierarchical piecewise exponential survival model to investigate the cancer risk for the tumour necrosis factor ("TNF")-inhibitor drug class. The Bayesian model was able to analyse the individual participant-level meta-data, take into account participant-level and possibly time-dependent covariates and model between study heterogeneity. Kaizar et al. [211] used the Bayesian hierarchical model to quantify the risk of suicidality for children who use antidepressants. Ibrahim et al. [212] developed a Bayesian meta-analytical sample size determination method for planning a phase II/III antidiabetic drug development programme.

4.4.3　Important considerations

While Bayesian methods are appealing, they can be computationally complex to implement. Care must be taken to check many aspects of the methodology (e.g. if MCMC methods are used, the convergence of the Markov chain, sensitivity to specific prior distributions and initial values should all be checked) [199]. It is recommended that, whenever the Bayesian methods are employed, expertise should be sought to ensure appropriate implementation.

Historically, computation time was an issue, but recent advances in software development (e.g. WinBUGS, SAS PROC MCMC, JAGS and especially Stan) have improved this situation.

Sensitivity analyses are particularly important for Bayesian analyses. While general advice for sensitivity analysis is given in section 4.9, we note one thing that is particularly important for Bayesian analysis. Any given Bayesian analysis may have several priors. Sensitivity analyses are required to check how influential the priors are. In addition, as when using other traditional statistical approaches, sensitivity analysis utilizing appropriate statistical models should also be performed.

4.5　Power

Summary of main points:

▶ Most meta-analyses for regulatory purposes analyse all relevant existing data at the time of the analysis and hence study power is used for descriptive purposes rather than planning purposes. In the regulatory setting, however, a prospectively-planned meta-analysis may be agreed between regulators and the sponsor. In this case power should be part of the protocol.

▶ A random-effects meta-analysis will generally will have less power than a fixed-effect meta-analysis because of the inclusion of the between-study variability.

▶ Tests of heterogeneity of the treatment effect across studies or within or across subgroups are likely to be less powerful than the test of the overall treatment effect.

▶ Tests of interactions or multiple subgroups have the same weaknesses regarding power and type I error in meta-analysis as in clinical trials.

The purpose of this section is to highlight important considerations regarding statistical power in the context of meta-analysis. It is not intended to give a synopsis of statistical power or formulas for power calculations.

The power of a meta-analysis is defined as the probability of rejecting the null hypothesis (at a significance level of α) when a specified alternative hypothesis is true. For this discussion we shall assume that the alternative hypothesis is that the true effect size between treatments is θ. Whereas power is an important planning concept used to determine study sample size for clinical trials, it may be less important prospectively in meta-analysis which, in most settings, analyses all relevant existing data at the time of the analysis. In the regulatory setting, however, a prospectively-planned meta-analysis in which power should be part of the protocol may be agreed on between regulators and the sponsor.

For example, if the parameter of interest is an OR and this is assumed to be common to all studies, then for any background event rate and an assumed relative risk – θ – the required number of events to yield a specified power to detect θ could be calculated and used to determine if a prospective meta-analysis were feasible. Similarly, in a non-inferiority setting, the number of events required to exclude a particular value of the relative risk could also be calculated.

More realistically, a single value θ may not be common to all studies, but rather there may be a distribution of study-specific θ_i between studies, with a between-study variability. If there is not a common θ across all studies then the overall treatment effect being estimated is determined by the way in which the individual study estimates are combined to obtain the overall estimate. The way in which the individual study estimates are combined may (but does not have to) incorporate the between-study variability. Thus, in a random-effects model, which incorporates the between-study variability in the standard error of the treatment effect, an assumption regarding the variability of θ^i would be needed to calculate power prior to conducting the meta-analysis.

In the context of meta-analysis there are a number of important points to keep in mind regarding power. Some of these points are derived from Hedges & Pigott [213, 214].

▶ A random-effects meta-analysis will generally have less power than a fixed-effect meta-analysis, due to the inclusion of the between-study variability of θ_i in the analysis (though this extra power will come with an increase in type I error). For example, a meta-analysis may include a study with a large treatment effect but with relatively few events. If the weights are the inverse of the variances then this study would be given relatively more weight in the random-effects model than in a fixed-effect model, which would result in a larger effect size and possibly greater power. The point is that the parameter being estimated will depend on the choice of analytical model and hence the realized ability of a meta-analysis to separate from the null hypothesis will depend on the choice of analytical method.

▶ The test of heterogeneity of the treatment effect across studies is a test of interactions and is likely to be less powerful than the test of the overall treatment effect, particularly if the interaction is one of degree in the treatment effect rather than the opposite direction. Again, this does not have to be the case. For example, the treatment effect over all studies could be zero but the variability of the treatment effect across studies could be large.

▶ Similarly, the test of differential treatment effects across subgroups (whether categorized by type of study or by a factor within studies) is likely to be less powerful than the test of the overall treatment effect, particularly if the interaction is one of degree in the treatment effect rather than the opposite direction. Because of the reduced power, the lack of significance in a subgroup analysis should not be interpreted as conclusive evidence that the treatment effect does not differ across subgroups.

▶ In a subgroup analysis, the size of the interaction effect could be larger than the average overall treatment effect, thereby yielding greater power for the interaction test. It should be stressed that a statistically significant interaction, particularly in the absence of an overall treatment effect, should be interpreted as an exploratory finding. Even if testing this interaction was the primary objective of the meta-analysis, there would still be concerns related to the comparability of treatment arms within subgroups (See section 4.8.1).

▶ In the absence of a significant overall treatment effect, the point estimate and the 95% CI are better measures in interpreting the results than is post hoc power. It is recommended that the upper and lower confidence bounds be given greater weight than post hoc power.

4.6 Missing data

Summary of main points:

▶ In a meta-analysis, missing data can result from missing entire studies, missing an outcome (or statistic) of interest and missing data from some individuals within an RCT.

▶ All data analysts face the problem of missing data. This section provides an overview of missing data issues that can occur in a meta-analysis of RCTs and discusses common approaches for handling them. Specific considerations for safety outcomes are identified.

4.6.1   Overview of missing data

In the context of systematic reviews or meta-analyses, potential sources of missing data can be classified into the following three main categories: (i) entire studies are missing from a review; (ii) an outcome of interest to the review is missing from an individual study; and (iii) data are missing from some individuals within an RCT.

(i) Entire studies are missing from a review:

Missing whole studies is not an issue unique to meta-analyses of safety data. Common examples of missing studies include unpublished studies or studies published in a foreign language. When entire studies are not published, there might be a major threat to the validity of meta-analyses when attempting to evaluate the totality of available evidence. The same is true for meta-analyses of safety data, as unpublished trials may be a better source of information on AEs than published trials [215]. A major concern about meta-analyses is the possibility of publication bias – i.e. the selective publication of studies based on the nature of their findings. A comprehensive search strategy should be used to help identify a wide range of published and unpublished studies to minimize publication bias. Section 3.8 discussed this point in more detail.

Funnel plots [132] are a means of detecting potential publication bias. Section 3.8.4 provides a detailed description of a funnel plot, including the symmetrical funnel plot in the absence of bias and the asymmetrical funnel plot in the presence of bias.

In analyses based on published studies, publication bias can result from the failure to include unpublished data combined with a preference for academic journals to publish studies based on the direction or statistical significance of results (e.g. [216]). Studies with positive results are often more likely to be referenced in subsequent publications, which may affect the studies selected if the search strategy is not comprehensive [217]. Note that the problem of publication bias has typically been raised in the context of efficacy analyses. Nonetheless, the potential for studies reporting relevant safety data to be missing should not be ignored.

Study results can also influence the likelihood that the study will be reported in multiple publications, and so care must be taken that duplicate data are not included in the meta-analysis [6], [218]. Due to the increased likelihood of multiple publications for a single study with positive results, this may lead to overestimation of the treatment effect. However, the aim should be to include all trials relevant to the study hypothesis irrespective of the single trial result.

ii) An outcome of interest to the review is missing from an individual study:

Missing outcome data from RCTs can lead to greater uncertainty and possible bias in estimating the safety of an experimental treatment. There are three main reasons that would lead to missing outcome data.

One reason for missing outcomes in a meta-analysis of RCTs of safety data is incomplete reporting. Many studies collect a range of outcome measures but do not report them all. If the decision as to which results to report from an RCT is influenced by the findings, then this would probably bias the results of the meta-analysis [219, 220]. Incomplete reporting can be especially problematic for the meta-analysis of safety data. For example, reports of clinical trials usually emphasize efficacy outcomes, resulting in a less thorough documentation of AEs [126, 127, 221, 222]. Some studies might not provide any information on AEs. Some studies might report only AEs considered to be drug-related by the original investigators. Sometimes the manuscript will restrict reporting to more frequently occurring events (e.g. "we only reported events with >=2% incidence in the treated group"). One of the problems with a meta-analysis for safety data is that events may be missing for many reasons, and it is often difficult for authors of a review to ascertain the reason for incomplete reporting of AEs. The possibility of inconsistency in rules for excluding data from the final report can create a much bigger problem when trying to correct for missing data analytically.

A second reason for missing outcome data comes from inconsistency in the reporting of summary statistics in the original studies. The meta-analysts often cannot compute a summary statistics for an outcome, in a format (such as ORs, RRs, HRs) appropriate for inclusion in a meta-analysis, from the information given in a study. For instance, studies may fail to report the sample size of each individual intervention group, the number of events, measures of variability (such as standard error or CIs), participants' follow-up periods, and/or important details about time-to-event outcomes.

A third reason for missing outcome data may arise from inappropriate analyses in the original studies. For example, a particular trial report may not make clear the method of handling missing data used to calculate the treatment effect. The meta-analysis could then be combining estimates that have been obtained using different methods of analysis, jeopardizing the validity of the meta-analysis.

In general, identification of missing outcome data should not be used as a reason to exclude a study from a systematic review or a meta-analysis. Whenever possible, a meta-analyst should contact the original investigators to seek the missing information on specific outcomes, analyses or methods of handling missing data that may not be clear in the final report.

(iii) Data are missing from some individuals within an RCT:

Unanalysed participant data might result when an intention-to-treat analysis is not conducted (i.e. when not all randomized participants are included in the analyses). Other examples include nonresponse, failure to record participant outcomes, and participant attrition. Another aspect of data that may be missing is pertinent information on risk factors for the outcome of interest that would allow evaluation of potential imbalance between the drug and placebo groups resulting from differential dropout of trial participants.

4.6.2   Commonly used methods for handling missing data in a meta-analysis

Missing outcome data are a common threat to the validity of the results from RCTs which, if not analysed appropriately, can lead to misleading treatment effect estimates. Many statistical approaches have been developed to deal with missing data on individuals within a RCT, including: i) the last observation carried forward technique, ii) least squares analysis, iii) imputation methods, and iv) likelihood-based approaches [223]. Advanced methodologies, such as multiple imputation, pattern mixture models and full likelihood analysis of available data, require that there be detailed data for each participant. Thus, implementation of advanced methodologies becomes challenging in a meta-analysis of summary data from RCTs since the summary data are often obtained from published reports from which limited information may be available for each participant.

Studies with missing outcome data also threaten the validity of any meta-analysis that includes them. The Cochrane Handbook [6] and National Institute for Health and Care Excellence [224, 225] provide recommendations on how missing data should be handled within a meta-analysis in an attempt to account for this potential bias and uncertainty around treatment estimates induced by missing data. These recommendations include:

1.   Making a judgement as to the level of bias due to missing data in each individual trial.

2.   Exploring the impact of this potential bias.

3.   Carrying out a number of sensitivity analyses by making different assumptions about the missing outcomes.

Two helpful papers that present how to use different imputation strategies or a statistical model using a Bayesian statistical approach to account for bias and to quantify uncertainty in treatment effect estimates induced by missing data are those of Turner et al. and Higgins et al. [226, 227].

In summary, missing data in a meta-analysis of RCTs occur in the form of missing studies from a review, missing or insufficient summary data, or missing data for some individuals within an RCT. When entire studies are missing from a review, identification of publication bias and checking of the sensitivity of results to publication bias should be considered. When an outcome of interest to the meta-analysis is missing from an RCT or when missing data issues occur for some individuals within a RCT, the aforementioned methodologies should be considered to handle the missing data. Further, the potential impact of the missing data on the findings of the review should be clearly addressed. When a meta-analysis is based on summary information from published papers, the amount of missing data and the way in which the data were handled by the author may be factors for consideration in assessing the methodological quality of individual trials. Whenever possible, the original authors should be contacted for missing data or to answer questions about the way the missing data were handled.

4.7 Multiplicity in meta-analysis and cumulative meta-analysis

Summary of main points:

▶ Cumulative meta-analysis involves a prospective plan for multiple testing over time as the new data from one or more studies accumulate.

▶ A type I error rate could be substantially increased due to multiple testing (e.g. over multiple doses, outcomes, subgroups, time periods, effect measures, looks at accumulating data) through meta-analysis.

▶ If the primary outcome measure is not predefined, the false positive rate could be further increased due to data-driven selection of the outcome measure of interest.

▶ The problem of an increased false positive rate due to multiple testing is largely ignored due to a lack of practical and satisfactory solutions.

▶ Most approaches require knowing the number of trials and/or sample size within the trials in advance, which is usually not the case. Uncertainty exists even when cumulative meta-analyses are planned during programme planning since these are often subject to change (especially in the case of adaptive trials).

▶ Bayesian methods generally allow probability statements to be made directly regarding quantities of interest, while uncertainty on other nuisance parameters is automatically accounted for in the analysis.

A type I error rate, the chance of a false positive finding (concluding that there is a treatment difference when in fact there is no difference),with respect to safety (or efficacy) could be substantially increased due to multiple testing (over multiple doses, outcomes, subgroups, time periods, effect measures, analyses of accumulating data, etc.) through meta-analysis. One situation in which multiplicity arises is in the context of cumulative meta-analysis. Cumulative meta-analysis is a meta-analysis in which studies are added one at a time in a specified order (e.g. according to date of study completion or publication) and the results are summarized as each new study is added. It is useful to think of a cumulative meta-analysis as a series of meta-analyses that are planned prospectively, with new studies being added to the body of evidence as they are completed. The cumulative meta-analysis should include a formal plan that specifies how the statistical significance level will be adjusted as the new data from one or more studies accumulate. The multiplicity issues in cumulative meta-analysis, where the focus is on addressing the same question (one endpoint) over time, become magnified when there are multiple endpoints.

In their investigation of a random sample of systematic reviews drawn from the Cochrane library, Biester & Lange [228] found that the number of outcomes varied from 1 to 35 with the median number of outcomes around 6. In addition, they have noted that only 47% of the cumulative meta-analyses had tried to make a distinction between primary and secondary outcomes.

If the primary outcome measure is not predefined, the false positive rate could be further increased due to data-driven selection of the outcome measure of interest. For example, in an ongoing series of studies, the primary safety outcome measure may be defined after some trials have been completed and its definition could be post hoc and driven by the observations from the completed trials. Here the results would be at best exploratory.

In the early cumulative meta-analysis papers, the problem of an increased false positive rate due to multiple testing was largely ignored [229-231]. The practice seems to have continued, as evidenced by the investigation of Biester & Lange, in which they found that only 4% of the authors of the cumulative meta-analysis papers made any statement about multiplicity adjustment with 2% having made an adjustment. They concluded that multiplicity is a commonly neglected problem in cumulative meta-analysis [228].

Several authors have proposed methods to control the false positive rate. Sequential approaches to control the false positive rate have been discussed by some authors [232-234]. Whitehead proposed use of triangle boundaries in the context of a drug development programme where a set number of interim analyses would be planned prospectively to determine as soon as possible whether the treatment was efficacious. Pogue & Yusuf [233] considered application of conventional group sequential methods such as O'Brien-Fleming type alpha-spending approach [235, 236]. In van der Tweel & Bollen's article [234], performance characteristics of these approaches (named by the authors as sequential meta-analysis for the triangle boundary, and trial sequential analysis for the O'Brien-Fleming type boundary) are compared. These approaches are criticized for their requirement of knowing the number of trials and/or sample size within the trials. Usually uncertainty exists even when cumulative meta-analyses are planned during programme planning since these are often subject to change (especially in case of adaptive trials). Further developments and discussion on sequential analysis can be found in papers by Kulinskaya & Wood, Imberger et al., Miladinovic et al., Higgins et al., Thorlund et al., Brok et al., and Wetterslev et al. [237-243].

In some clinical development programmes, meta-analyses are performed repeatedly and additional safety studies may be initiated if available data are not conclusive. One example is the cardiovascular outcome study required by the FDA for diabetes drugs. Jennison & Turnbull [244] apply the P value combination approach to the cumulative meta-analyses to address the adaptive nature of these kinds of programmes. Adaptive and repeated safety cumulative meta-analyses present even more challenges from a multiplicity viewpoint. The frequentist approach (revised versions of the Fisher's P value combination test) and Bayesian approaches suggested by Quan et al. [245] can be applicable and useful in the control of type I error rate.

Lan et al. [246] suggest an approach based on the law of iterated logarithms (LIL) that penalizes the z-value of the test statistic to account for multiple tests in a cumulative meta-analysis of a continuous endpoint that is either planned prospectively or examined retrospectively. The method also accounts for estimation of heterogeneity in treatment effects across studies. Hu et al. extend this method for the analysis of binary outcomes of relative risk, OR, or RDs. Their methods are flexible so that analyses can take place at variable time points and leave the maximum information unspecified. However, one should be aware that there could be an extensive loss of power from use of the LIL approach in scenarios where the between-study heterogeneity is reasonably small and the maximum information is pre-specified [247]. For example, use of the LIL approach for within-trial monitoring is not recommended when participants are not expected to be extremely diversified. In these scenarios, conventional approaches such as alpha-spending function can control type I error rate and are more powerful than the LIL approach. In scenarios with high between-study heterogeneity or unspecified maximum information, for which the LIL approach has been developed, it is less clear how conservative the LIL approach is compared to others since other commonly-used methods may not protect the type I error rate. It is recommended by Hu et al. to use simulation to determine the appropriate adjustment factor in order to control the type I error rate and also achieve the optimal power.

While these approaches may help to control the false positive rate at a nominal level, there are limitations, such as the requirement of knowing the number and size of the trials for the sequential approaches or reduced power to detect a difference for the LIL approach. In addition, for a cumulative meta-analysis of a safety outcome, there may be an argument, especially from a regulatory standpoint, that a multiplicity adjustment is not acceptable since the emphasis is on the power to detect a potential safety signal. If no multiplicity adjustment is implemented, interpretation of potential positive findings from such a cumulative meta-analysis needs to be carefully assessed in the context of possible inflation in false positive findings. In such instances, the focus should be placed on estimation instead of inference and the evidence may be considered hypothesis-generating. It should be noted that nominal vs. adjusted P values could lead to different conclusions. All of these considerations take on even more importance when the endpoint is a very severe AE, such as mortality.

According to Lau et al. [248], cumulative meta-analysis is most naturally interpreted in the Bayesian framework. In this framework, the knowledge available before the current data arrive is incorporated into the prior distribution and the knowledge available after the current data are processed is expressed by the posterior distribution. This posterior distribution then becomes the new prior distribution when more data arrive. Bayesian analysis deals with multiplicity adjustment solely through the assignment of prior probabilities to models or hypotheses. Bayesian methods generally allow probability statements to be made directly regarding quantities of interest, while uncertainty on other nuisance parameters is automatically accounted for in the analysis. Here conclusions (credible intervals) are expressed as probabilistic statements about beliefs rather than as definite statements about hypotheses. A novel Bayesian sample size determination method for sequential meta-analysis controlling for multiplicity in the context of evaluating cardiovascular risk for anti-diabetic drugs has been proposed [249].

As mentioned in section 4.4, the subjectivity associated with picking a prior distribution is considered to be a negative feature by some. Historically, critics of the Bayesian paradigm have focused their criticisms on the choice of the prior distribution. These criticisms had some validity in the sense that there is no unique way of choosing prior distributions, but the contribution from Jeffreys on non-informative priors had somewhat eased the criticism [250]. More recently, theoretical developments on robustness and sensitivity analysis have also provided a sounder basis for Bayesian analysis when it is faced with incomplete prior information. In addition, introduction of hierarchical modelling has allowed for pushing the prior selection to higher levels, with an observed decrease in the influence on the resulting inference.

Bender et al. [251] have offered some suggestions for dealing with the problem of multiplicity. They have concluded that "there is no simple or completely satisfactory solution to the problem of multiple comparisons in systematic reviews. It is however, an issue that requires recognition. Authors and users of reviews need to be careful about multiplicity when presenting, interpreting and using reviews that contain or are based on numerous statistical analyses."

Because of the lack of a satisfactory solution to this multiplicity problem, some use cumulative meta-analysis only as an exploratory tool and simply report the number of analyses performed without attempting to adjust for multiplicity. Thus, one of the approaches to multiplicity for cumulative meta-analysis can be analogous to that for conventional safety analysis. In conventional safety analysis, nominal P values from hypothesis-testing are usually provided without adjustment for a limited number of pre-specified outcomes.

4.8 Heterogeneity

Summary of main points:

▶ Heterogeneity can generally be classified as clinical, methodological or statistical. Clinical and methodological heterogeneity do not necessarily result in statistical heterogeneity. Low overall statistical heterogeneity does not necessarily mean absence of difference in treatment effects across specific subgroups of patients or subsets of studies.

▶ The main ways of detecting or estimating statistical heterogeneity are graphical, such as forest plots, or statistical (e.g. Cochran's Q, I^2, test of interaction).

▶ When heterogeneity of results is identified, it is valuable to understand and study the clinical or methodological factors, if any, that are associated with that heterogeneity, as these associations may indicate that those specific factors modify the impact of treatment.

▶ Subgroup analysis and meta-regression are ways of exploring heterogeneous results, or answering specific questions about specific patient or study characteristics.

▶ Whenever possible, potential sources of clinical or methodological heterogeneity that might lead to statistical heterogeneity should be specified in the protocol and ideally only a few characteristics will be investigated

▶ Meta-regression and subgroup analyses can result in misleading conclusions even if undertaken with care. Conclusions from subgroup analyses and meta-regression should be drawn cautiously.

Heterogeneity, in its broadest sense, refers to differences between studies and/or study results. Heterogeneity can generally be classified in three ways: clinical heterogeneity, methodological heterogeneity and statistical heterogeneity [191, 252]. Clinical heterogeneity refers to differences between trials in their participant selection (e.g. disease conditions under investigation, eligibility criteria, participant characteristics, or geographical differences), interventions (e.g. duration, dosing, type of control) and outcomes (e.g. definitions of endpoints, follow-up duration, cut-off points for scales). Methodological heterogeneity refers to the differences in study design (e.g. the mechanism of randomization) and in study conduct (e.g. allocation concealment, blinding, extent and handling of withdrawals and loss to follow-up, or analysis methods). Decisions about what constitutes clinical heterogeneity and methodological heterogeneity do not involve any calculation and are based on judgement.

On the other hand, statistical heterogeneity represents a notion that individual studies may have results that are not numerically consistent with each other, and the variation is more than what is expected on the basis of sampling variability alone. Statistical heterogeneity may be caused by known clinical and methodological differences between trials, by unknown trial (clinical or methodological) characteristics, or it may be due to chance. Figure 4.1 illustrates the variability of treatment effects for a binary outcome from study to study in the two cases of limited (left side) and large (right side) variation across studies. How these different types of variation affect the choice of statistical model is described in more detail in section 4.3.

Figure 4.1 Effect size variation across studies

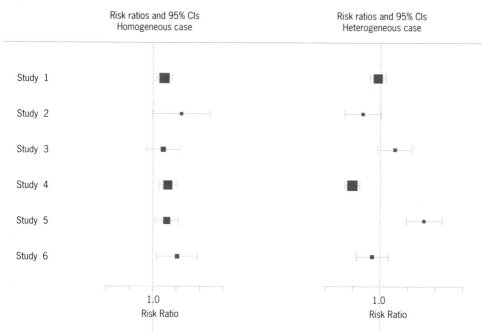

Source: Crowe, BJ created for CIOMS X (2016).

The main ways of detecting or estimating statistical heterogeneity are graphical, such as forest plots (see Figures 4.1 and 4.2) or statistical (e.g. Cochran's Q, I^2, test of interaction). See section 4.3.4 for more on Q and I^2. Visually, the results on the left side of Figure 4.1 are quite consistent, in contrast with the impression from the graph on the right which suggests that the studies, for whatever reason (possibly including bias), may not be estimating the same quantity. The results on the right should serve as a prompt to do a thorough job of trying to understand the reasons for the heterogeneity of results (though this could be difficult with so few studies).

It is important to be mindful that absence of statistical heterogeneity does not necessarily mean absence of clinical heterogeneity or the true absence of differential treatment effects. Furthermore, clinical heterogeneity may not always result in statistical heterogeneity. In some situations consistency of results across diverse studies may represent robust, generalizable treatment effects.

It is often assumed that it is inappropriate to combine studies that have quite different baseline event rates. Differences in baseline (control) rates, however, do not necessarily translate into large differences in treatment effect sizes across studies. Furthermore, when treatment effects do appear heterogeneous, it may still be possible to choose a metric/scale that leads to treatment effects that are sufficiently homogeneous to be interpretable. Risk differences tend to be more heterogeneous than ORs or relative risks [166], a point that is also made in an FDA draft guidance for industry on non-inferiority trials [253]. For binary outcomes, changing the scale from an absolute measure (like risk difference) to a relative measure, such as OR or relative risk, might reduce statistical heterogeneity and make the data sufficiently homogeneous to produce a meaningful combined estimate on that ratio scale. The combined result can then be converted (e.g. from an OR to a RD) to help with clinical interpretability. Because the constant OR model implies that the effect size must vary on the RD scale, a decision is needed as to whether to estimate the baseline (control) event rate from external data or from the data included in the actual meta-analysis. These two approaches have different implications for the analysis, especially variance estimation [167].

Strategies for addressing statistical heterogeneity include checking again that data are correct, not doing a meta-analysis at all, as in the case that quoting an overall average could be misleading (e.g. when effect sizes vary dramatically on either side of the null), exploring heterogeneity (e.g. via subgroup analyses and meta-regression), changing the effect measure (see section 4.1) and excluding studies [6]. Because of the importance of exploring and understanding heterogeneity, the rest of this section focuses on subgroup analysis and meta-regression.

4.8.1　Subgroup analysis

Subgroup analyses involve splitting data into subgroups so that comparisons can be made between them. Analyses may be conducted for subgroups of studies (such as different geographical locations) or subgroups of participants (such as males and females). These analyses can be used to compare the mean effect sizes between different subgroups. They may be done as a way of answering specific questions about particular participant groups, types of intervention or types of studies, or as a way of investigating heterogeneous results.

We first consider subgroups of studies. Suppose a meta-analysis was performed to assess the impact of a drug on lowering cholesterol and several studies were carried out in Europe and in the USA. It was postulated that the treatment effect would be different in Europe compared with the USA. Several methods (both fixed-effect and random-effects) could be used to compare the two subgroups. Some of these amount to study-level versions of z-tests (for two subgroups) and analysis of variance (ANOVA), if there are more than two subgroups to compare. For example, the subgroup analysis could proceed by first using meta-analysis techniques to calculate an overall mean treatment effect (with standard error) for the European studies and another for the American studies. Then a z-test could be used to test whether the mean treatment effects differ significantly between the groups and a difference (between the two subgroup mean treatment effects) could be calculated (with its standard error). Interested readers may check Borenstein et al. [4] and Deeks et al. [254] for further information on methods of estimating the difference in treatment effects between subgroups of studies and assess statistical heterogeneity between these subgroups.

Subgroup analyses of subsets of participants within studies are uncommon in systematic reviews of the literature because sufficient details about separate participant types are seldom published. When subgroup-specific results are presented (e.g. treatment effects in older and younger subjects are reported separately), then the subgroup-specific treatment effect estimates may be combined using meta-analysis techniques, keeping in mind the caveats discussed in section 4.8.3.

In contrast, if IPD are available, a substantial number of analysis methods are available. Methods can be broadly classified as those that analyse each study separately and then combine effect sizes using standard meta-analysis techniques (two-stage analysis) and those that analyse all of the data in one step (single-stage analysis) [4]. The latter methods allow for complex analyses, such as multilevel modelling, that can explore associations between intervention effects and participant-level or study-level characteristics. IPD permits estimating effects for subgroups of participants defined by participant-level characteristics. In general, it is more appropriate to conduct a single-stage analysis of the IPD, in which one incorporates terms for treatment, the covariate of interest (subgroup membership) and the interaction term, although it may also be helpful, descriptively, to produce separate summary treatment effect estimates within each subgroup. Note, however, that even using the single-stage analyses, it is straightforward to produce summary estimates derived from subgroups (subsets) of studies (e.g. studies with longer duration of follow-up vs. those with shorter duration of follow-up).

4.8.2 Meta-regression

Meta-regression is a form of regression analysis in which the unit of analysis is a study, not the IPD. It is an extension to subgroup analyses that allows the effect of continuous, as well as categorical, characteristics to be investigated and in principle allows the effects of multiple factors to be investigated simultaneously (although this is often not possible due to inadequate numbers of studies) [105].

The technique uses study-level summary data to explore the relationship between study characteristics (e.g. concealment of allocation, baseline risk, timing of the intervention) and study effect estimate (e.g. risk difference, log OR, or log RR). If there are few studies, even if there are many patients, meta-regression is unlikely to be scientifically useful. Meta-regression should generally not be considered when there are fewer than 10 studies in a meta-analysis [6].

Because meta-regression has study-level summary statistics as response and explanatory variables, it is important to weight each study in the regression and to select the appropriate model (fixed-effect vs. random-effects), though in most cases the random-effects model will be appropriate [255]. Many methods can be considered and we refer interested readers to papers such as references [4, 255, 256].

Meta-regression models rely on the summary results of published studies as well as summary estimates of participant characteristics. These summary results describe only between-study, and not between-participant, variation in the risk factors. For that reason, they are most useful for characteristics that differ across studies and that are shared by all participants in the same study.

If full IPD are available, a substantial number of analysis methods are available, as described in section 3.9.

When IPD are not available, many characteristics that might vary substantially among participants within a study can be summarized only at the level of the study (e.g. age). While these can be analysed at the study level, such analyses may give biased results. The problem is one of aggregating individuals' results and is variously known as aggregation bias, ecological bias or the ecological fallacy [139, 257, 258]. The difficulties with summary-level data for the detection of subgroup differences are not limited to ecological bias. Lambert et al., in a simulation study, point out that the summary-level analyses often have low statistical power to detect interactions (also known as effect modification) [140]. Similarly, Schmid et al. (2004) performed analyses of two datasets and showed that subgroup differences of interest were detected by IPD analyses but not by summary-level analyses [141]. In their first analysis, treatment effects were homogeneous across studies, and therefore meta-regression identified no interactions. Analysis of IPD from the same studies discovered an important modifier of treatment effect. Their second investigation found meta-regression to be effective for detecting treatment interactions with study-level factors in meta-analyses with at least 10 studies, with heterogeneous treatment effects or significant overall treatment effects.

4.8.3 General considerations for subgroup analysis and meta-regression

Whenever possible, potential sources of clinical or methodological diversity that might lead to statistical heterogeneity should be specified in the protocol. Pre-specifying characteristics reduces the likelihood of spurious findings by limiting the number of factors to analyse and preventing knowledge of the studies' results from influencing the choice of factors to be analysed. If more than one or two characteristics are investigated it may be sensible to adjust the level of significance to account for making multiple comparisons [6, section 9.6.5.3]. (See section 4.7 for more information on multiplicity.) Characteristics to be investigated should be clinically plausible and supported by other external or indirect evidence, if they are to be convincing.

While pre-specification of characteristics is recommended, in doing the qualitative synthesis of studies, reviewers may identify factors that they did not think of in advance. Such characteristics can be analysed, but it should be made clear when reporting results that they were not pre-specified. Analyses of characteristics defined *a posteriori* (also known as post hoc) are those that are guided by the data. Typically, they are those suggested only after preliminary analysis. Such analyses are potentially a form of data dredging [259, 260] and they may result in uncontrolled type I error [259-261] and are therefore subject to potential bias.

Caution should be exercised when characterizing the individual study attributes solely on the basis of the individual protocol specifications. In practice, for pragmatic reasons, studies have often deviated from the original plan. An effort should be made to confirm that the conduct of each study reflects the protocol specifications [9, 48].

Meta-regression and subgroup analyses can result in misleading conclusions even if undertaken with care. Subgroup analyses and meta-regressions are observational in their nature. Hence, they suffer the limitations of any observational investigation, including possible bias through confounding by other study-level (or participant-level) characteristics. Observed subgroup differences (even within-study) can sometimes be confounded because the comparability afforded to the main study groups might not necessarily be carried over to subgroups, potentially creating an imbalance in important participant attributes between these groups [48]. For instance, suppose gender subgroups are of particular interest. Although gender might be equally distributed between the drug and comparator groups due to randomization, if gender is associated with age in the study population, age may not be equally distributed between men and women. If age also modifies drug risk, then observed differences in adverse treatment effects between men and women might be caused by a difference in the distribution of age between the two subgroups.

Since different subgroups are likely to contain different amounts of information and thus differ in their abilities to detect effects, it is extremely misleading simply to compare the statistical significance of the results. An additional caveat is needed in performing such analyses. In some situations, an imbalance in covariates at baseline may be introduced due to differential dropout in the drug and control groups, especially in subgroups because of the smaller numbers. Even if data on the known and measured imbalanced factors are available, the distribution and potential imbalance of unmeasured pertinent risk factors in study subgroups would remain unknown, with unpredictable impact on the study findings [48].

4.9 Sensitivity analysis

Summary of main points:

▶ Sensitivity analysis is an approach to investigating how the decisions and assumptions from a meta-analysis influence the main findings and how robust the results are under a variety of decisions and assumptions.

▶ Sensitivity analysis should be performed to reflect the decisions made at all stages of a meta-analysis and should always be performed to assess the robustness of combined estimates.

▷ Some sensitivity analyses can be pre-specified in the study protocol, but many concerns suitable for sensitivity analysis are identified only during the review process where the individual peculiarities of the studies under investigation are identified.

Sensitivity analysis is an approach to investigating how the decisions and assumptions from a meta-analysis influence the main findings and how robust the results are under a variety of decisions and assumptions. For example, if the eligibility of some studies in the meta-analysis is dubious because they do not contain full details, sensitivity analysis may involve undertaking the meta-analysis twice: first, including all studies and second, only including those that are definitely known to be eligible. A sensitivity analysis asks the question, "Are the findings robust with respect to the decisions made in the process of obtaining them?" Various experts have argued that sensitivity analysis should be performed to reflect the decisions made at all stages of a meta-analysis [262] and always be performed to assess the robustness of combined estimates [263].

Planning of sensitivity analysis should start at an early stage. Investigators should identify important decisions and assumptions for sensitivity analysis, such as:

▷ The effect of including certain types of excluded studies, or of excluding certain types of included studies;

▷ How the combined estimates are affected by individual factors contributing to risk of bias, such as use of blinding, concealment of allocation, objective ascertainment of outcomes;

▷ Whether results derived from different effect measures (e.g. relative risk and risk difference) agree;

▷ Whether results from a fixed-effect model agree with those from a random-effects model, or different forms of a fixed-effect or random-effects model agree;

▷ How different approaches for handling missing data, zero cells, and incomplete data reporting affect the results

Sensitivity to the distributional assumptions can be assessed by assuming different distributions for the study effects and comparing subsequent inferences. For example, the analyst may assume that the underlying study effects arise from a Student-t distribution, thereby permitting heavier tails than those arising from a Normal distribution.

Some sensitivity analyses can be pre-specified in the study protocol, but many issues suitable for sensitivity analysis are identified only during the review process where the individual peculiarities of the studies under investigation are identified. In reporting, such post hoc analyses should be clearly identified as such.

When results of a fixed-effect model and a random-effects model disagree, it is important to try to understand the nature of, and the reasons for, that disagreement. If the only difference is in terms of precision, and the point estimates are similar, then it is useful to explore sources of heterogeneity (see section 4.8 on heterogeneity). In these situations, the difference in precision is likely to have arisen from heterogeneity of the within-study effects, with variation in opposite directions that happens to "balance out". If the point estimates disagree, that could be because small studies are showing systematically different results from larger studies. (In the random-effects models, the small studies are typically weighted more heavily). If so, are there characteristics of the small studies, or the populations enrolled in those studies, that make them systematically different from the larger studies?

When sensitivity analyses show that the overall result and conclusions are not affected by the different decisions that could be made during the review process, the results of the review can be regarded with a higher degree of certainty. Where sensitivity analyses identify particular decisions or missing information that greatly influence the findings of the review, greater resources can be deployed to try and resolve uncertainties and obtain extra information, possibly through contacting trial authors and obtaining IPD. If this cannot be achieved, the results must be interpreted with an appropriate degree of caution. Such findings may generate proposals for further investigations and future research.

Sensitivity analyses are sometimes confused with subgroup analysis. In general, sensitivity analyses are concerned with the robustness of the primary results from methodological decisions, whereas subgroup analyses are concerned with exploring the treatment effect across specific study characteristics. Although some sensitivity analyses involve restricting the analysis to a subset of the totality of studies, the two methods differ in two ways. First, sensitivity analyses do not attempt to estimate the effect of the intervention in the group of studies removed from the analysis, whereas in subgroup analyses, estimates are produced for each subgroup. Second, in sensitivity analyses, informal comparisons are made between different ways of estimating the same thing, whereas in subgroup analyses, formal statistical comparisons are made across the subgroups with the explicit objective of assessing whether the factor being examined might modify the effect of treatment. In principle, however, both approaches have the common goal of assessing robustness of findings across a range of approaches to the analyses.

4.10 Reporting for meta-analysis

Summary of main points:

▶ Guidelines exist for the reporting of traditional literature-based meta-analysis.

▶ This section provides a modified checklist with a focus on important reporting elements in the context of regulatory setting for safety assessment. The checklist is given in Table 4.1 and includes four main sections: Introduction, Methods, Results and Interpretation. The checklist also specifies items that are unique to frequentist and Bayesian analyses.

In order to promote a consistent approach for meta-analysis, standardization of meta-analysis reporting is needed so that all the stakeholders (regulators, sponsors, investigators, etc.) can understand and interpret the evidence synthesis more easily. Standard reporting would also promote scientific rigor and provide transparency so that a meta-analysis could be replicated and verified by other investigators and stakeholders.

Because forest plots are such an important part of the display of study results, the next section is dedicated to them (see also section 4.8 which introduced the topic of forest plots in the context of estimating statistical heterogeneity).

4.10.1 The use of forest plots

Graphical displays of data from meta-analysis are widely utilized – especially forest plots, which have gradually developed over time into a fairly standard form [264]. The forest plot is very useful for showing the main features, and may also be useful even if an overall summary is not produced. The example of a forest plot shown in Figure 4.2 is annotated with some explanation of the features.

Figure 4.2 An example of a forest plot

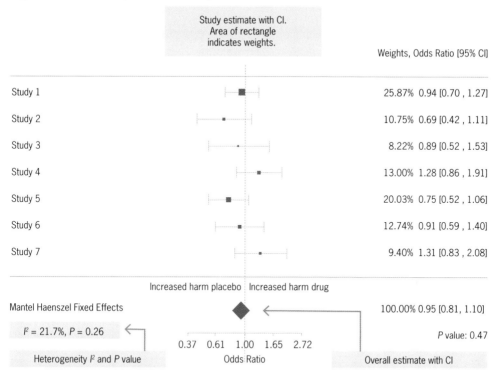

The horizontal lines show the CI around the effect estimate of the individual studies. At the point estimate a block is shown whose area is proportional to the amount of information (the weight is usually used) in that trial. The vertical line is drawn at the null value (no difference between the treatments) while the diamond is drawn around the overall summary, centred on the best estimate of the average effect across studies. The width of the diamond is an indicator of the CI for the summary value.

The horizontal axis is often drawn on a log scale when the effect estimate is a relative measure, like OR, RR or hazard ratio. When this is the case, the CIs are symmetric around the point estimate; otherwise they would be asymmetric. Details of the history and functions of forest plots are given in Lewis & Clarke [264].

4.10.2 Checklist for reporting

Guidelines are available for the reporting of traditional, literature-based meta-analysis. A guideline for reporting Meta-analysis of Observational Studies in Epidemiology (MOOSE) was published in 2000 [265]. In 2009, the Preferred Reporting Items for Systematic Reviews and Meta-Analyses (PRISMA) guidelines were published [18, 266]. These guidelines provide checklists of recommendations for reporting of meta-analyses of observational studies and RCTs, respectively. The checklists include recommendations on background, search strategy, inclusion/exclusion criteria, methods, results, discussion and conclusions. In addition, PRISMA guidelines suggest a flow diagram to provide information about the numbers of RCTs identified, included, and excluded and the reasons for exclusion of studies. (See Figure 4.3 below for an example of a flow diagram.) Since the original PRISMA guidelines were published, several additional guidelines have been released. These include PRISMA for protocols [267, 268], network meta-analysis [20], for individual participant data [19], and, of note, PRISMA specifically for harms (PRISMA-harms) [269]. The PRISMA-harms checklist adds four items to the 2009 PRISMA checklist. Hammad and colleagues present an empirical assessment of adherence to the PRISMA guidelines for meta-analyses assessing harms. They also present a table of additional meta-analysis characteristics that should be described for meta-analyses of harms [270].

Figure 4.3 Flow diagram of exclusions of trials and participants

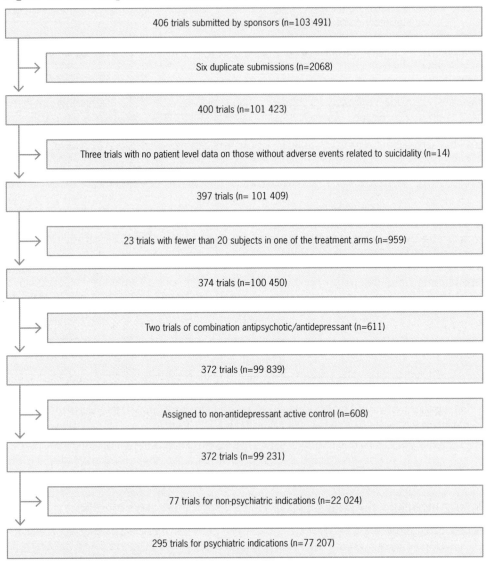

Source: Stone et al. Risk of suicidality in clinical trials of antidepressants in adults: analysis of proprietary data submitted to US Food and Drug Administration. BMJ, 2009, Fig.1 [271]. Used with permission of the publishers.

Based on the literature review, we modified the checklist of meta-analysis reporting with a focus on important reporting elements in the context of regulatory setting for safety assessment (see Table 4.1 below). The checklist includes four main sections: Introduction, Methods, Results and Interpretation. Each main section includes key elements of meta-analysis reporting related to that section and a brief description is also provided for each key element. The Introduction section includes items that are specific to the regulatory context and reasons for undertaking meta-analyses of harms, along with the meta-analysis objective(s). The Methods section focuses on aspects relative to the actual conduct of the evidence synthesis. The Results section relates to specific data summaries that should be presented. Finally, the Interpretation section discusses how meta-analysis results can be appropriately evaluated and utilized for decision-making.

In addition, we include specific aspects of Bayesian meta-analysis reporting [208]. The concepts considered in the process of a systematic review and meta-analysis (such as how to formulate a research question, or how to select studies) are completely relevant for any of meta-analysis, regardless of whether the analytical approach is frequentist or Bayesian [6, chapters 5-8]. However, there are important elements that are unique to Bayesian meta-analysis, which we highlight with asterisks in the first column of Table 4.1.

While Bayesian approaches offer many advantages in the context of using meta-analysis to assess drug safety, it is critically important to standardize the reporting process in the regulatory setting for reasons that go beyond the usual needs for transparency in general meta-analysis reporting. First, whereas numerous guidelines and considerable experience exist in the conduct and reporting of traditional frequentist analyses, the corresponding consensus regarding Bayesian analyses has only recently emerged among statisticians, and is largely unknown outside the statistical community. Second, Bayesian methods tend to be inherently more complex than classic frequentist analysis. There has been considerable variation in the reporting of Bayesian meta-analyses, so there is a need for the development of a list of items that should be reported when a Bayesian meta-analysis is performed. Third, the checklist can provide guidance to reviewers and readers who may not be familiar with Bayesian analyses to better understand such analyses. Finally, since the terminology tends to differ between a Bayesian and a traditional analysis, standardized reporting promotes the use of similar terminology and provides clear distinctions whenever a Bayesian meta-analysis is reported.

A few guidelines have been published in describing the important elements for reporting Bayesian analyses. Lang & Secic provided the following fundamental elements for Bayesian reporting [272]:

1. Report the pre-trial probabilities of certain hypotheses with respect to a treatment effect and specify how they were determined;

2. Report the post-trial probabilities and the corresponding intervals;

3. Interpret the post-trial probabilities.

Similar advice is provided in the *Annals of Internal Medicine's* instructions to authors of manuscripts using Bayesian methods to conduct data analyses. The Bayesian Standards in Science (BaSiS) group [273] developed a set of standards for reporting of Bayesian analyses in the scientific literature. Sung et al. [274] generated a set of seven items that experts believe to be most important when reporting a Bayesian analysis for scientific publications. A Bayesian checklist proposed by Spiegelhalter et al. [275] provided a solid foundation for what should be reported in a Bayesian analysis. Those authors also provided numerous examples in the book using the Bayesian checklist for reporting.

Table 4.1 Checklist for meta-analysis reporting, including Bayesian meta-analysis reporting

Item number	Important elements for reporting meta-analysis	What to consider in a frequentist framework	What to consider in a Bayesian framework
Introduction			
1	Introduction and background	Reasons for undertaking the meta-analysis and regulatory context if applicable; the intervention to be investigated with respect to the relevant population; brief overview of what is known about the state of evidence for the safety issue to be evaluated.	
2	Aim of the meta-analysis	Research questions and objectives of the meta-analysis.	
Methods			
3	Prospective meta-analysis?	Find out whether a protocol existed before data collection or analysis (and, if so, where it can be accessed)?	Find out whether a protocol existed before data collection or analysis (and, if so, where it can be accessed)? Find out whether the prior was constructed before data collection and analysis?
4	Outcome	Define the outcomes (e.g. MedDRA SMQ xyz narrow, MedDRA version) and whether the AE definitions are the same across studies. Describe the length of the assessment period for AEs in the component studies (e.g. duration of therapy + 30 days); criteria for combinability of subjects, treatments (doses), outcomes and lengths of follow-up; and procedures for assessment of outcomes (e.g. blinded to treatment assignment). Distinguish between studies designed to assess the outcome (i.e. whether the AEs under study were predefined endpoints) and studies in which the outcome was assessed after study completion; whether the AEs were specifically elicited or reported spontaneously. Ascertain whether the AEs reported in the paper were only those that the investigators considered to be drug-related. Describe adjudication procedure(s) and charter for clinical expert committees.	

Item number	Important elements for reporting meta-analysis	What to consider in a frequentist framework	What to consider in a Bayesian framework
5	Eligibility criteria and study selection	Specify study characteristics used as criteria for eligibility (e.g. PICOS, length of follow-up), giving rationale; state the process for selecting studies; describe efforts to avoid double-counting of component studies (i.e. studies reported in more than one publication); disclose whether studies were excluded because they reported none of the AEs of interest; and describe any enrichment strategies that may have been used to define populations in the original studies (e.g. selecting individuals at high risk of cardiovascular disease). Specify whether the protocols (and protocol amendments) of each study were accessed and reviewed to examine homogeneity of the nuance of study design among trials. Describe whether an effort was made to confirm studies were conducted per protocol regarding the characteristics of patients recruited.	
6	Search strategy and information sources	Present full electronic search strategy for at least one database, including any limits used, such that it could be repeated. Describe all information sources (e.g. databases with dates of coverage, contact with study authors to identify additional studies) in the search and date last searched.	
7	Data extraction process	Describe method of data extraction from reports (e.g. piloted forms, independently, in duplicate) and any processes for obtaining and confirming data from investigators.	
8	Data items and risk metrics	List and define all variables for which data were sought (e.g. PICOS) and any assumptions, simplifications or conversions (e.g. between risk metrics) made.	
9	Risk of bias in individual studies and across studies	Describe any assessment of risk of bias in individual studies (including study-level and outcome–level) and across studies. For example, consider the extent of loss to follow-up measured and reported in the component studies and, if so, how/whether this was used in any data synthesis.	
10	Effect measure(s)	Define the selected effect measure(s) (e.g. RD, OR or RR) and whether some transformations between various measures were calculated.	
11	Analysis population	For example, intention-to-treat, as-treated or per-protocol. Different studies may have different analytical populations. Present demographic data for the meta-analysis population and an overview of the number of patients per drug. See Table 4.2 below for an example of the latter.	

Item number	Important elements for reporting meta-analysis	What to consider in a frequentist framework	What to consider in a Bayesian framework
12	Specifying statistical model for evidence synthesis	Structure of levels of model; choice of fixed-effect vs. random-effects models and rationale for choice; choice of specific weighting schemes.	Choice of prior (and hyper prior if hierarchical modelling is used); distribution and rationale for choice; alternative priors for the purpose of sensitivity analysis should be explicitly specified.
13	Subgroup analysis	Consider whether subgroup analyses (for the meta-analysis) were pre-specified; address the potential for imbalance of baseline covariates between treatment groups within subgroups.	
14	Zero events	Specifically mention how zero events were handled, if relevant.	
15	Model checks and sensitivity analysis	Consider approaches used to check model fit and to carry out any sensitivity analyses (e.g. handling of missing data, handling of sparse data, etc.)	Although model checks and sensitivity analysis are not unique to Bayesian analyses, the potential for the Bayesian result to be dependent on model assumptions is high.
16	Computation/software	Computational methods for generating inferences; software used and how it is validated if not commercially available.	Computational methods for generating posterior inferences; if MCMC is used, how convergence is checked; other relevant commands and options.
Results			
17	Study selection	Draw up a flowchart to show how the final studies were selected for inclusion in the primary analysis, providing numbers of studies being included, with reasons for exclusions of certain studies; in particular, note which studies were excluded only because they did not report AEs. Describe efforts to contact original study authors for additional information, and, if authors were contacted for these studies, did they respond? If so, which additional studies were included as a result of contacting authors?	

Item number	Important elements for reporting meta-analysis	What to consider in a frequentist framework	What to consider in a Bayesian framework
18	Study characteristics	For each study, present study characteristics for which data are extracted (e.g. study size, PICOS, follow-up period).	
19	Risk of bias within studies and across studies	Present results of any assessment of risk of bias within studies and across studies. Discuss (qualitatively) differences among protocols or study attributes that could have resulted in differences in study findings. These are attributes that might be utilized in a meta-regression, as appropriate. (e.g. differences in inclusion and exclusion criteria as well as design nuances that might result in recruiting high-/low-risk patients, duration of follow-up, location (North America/non-North America), setting (inpatient/outpatient), nature of comparator group(s) (e.g. presence of an active control arm or not), number of centres, sample size per trial, differences in screening at baseline, and exclusion of subpopulations such as placebo respondents (run-in periods), treatment-resistant patients, high-risk patients at baseline for AE, or patients with history of AE, and so on.	
20	Results of individual studies	Present summary data for each intervention group, and point estimates and confidence or credible intervals for the treatment effect in each study, ideally with a forest plot.	
21	Synthesis of results	Present results on overall treatment effect and CI, as well as measures of consistency.	Present overall treatment effect and credible interval, summaries (numerical and/or graphical) of the posterior distribution of study specific and overall model parameters, and other quantities of interest.
22	Additional analysis	Give results of any additional analyses, if done (e.g. sensitivity, subgroup or meta-regression).	
Interpretation			
23	Summary of evidence	Summarize the main findings of meta-analysis, including strength of evidence, as well as remaining uncertainties. Describe any assessment of possible causality.	
24	Sensitivity analysis	Include the impact of sensitivity analyses on the results and interpretation of analysis findings.	
25	Possible limitations of the analysis	Include a candid appraisal of all strengths and possible weaknesses of the analysis.	

Source: Created by CIOMS X (2016).

Many items, including items in Table 4.1, overlap with and should be considered as complementary to the established meta-analysis reporting guidelines such as the various PRISMA statements.

Table 4.2 Number of participants by drug, drug class and treatment assignment

Drug	Primary	Active control	Placebo
Selective serotonin reuptake inhibitors			
Citalopram	1928	733	1371
Escitalopram	2567	563	2604
Fluoxetine	9070	2418	7645
Fluvoxamine	2187	0	1828
Paroxetine	8728	1223	7005
Sertraline	5821	1129	5589
Duloxetine	6361	0	4172
Venlafaxine	5693	129	4054
Other modern antidepressants:			
Bupropion	6018	0	3887
Mirtazapine	1268	0	726
Nefazodone	3319	0	2173
Tricyclic antidepressants:			
Amitriptyline	0	625	627
Clomipramine	0	632	617
Desipramine	0	315	298
Dosulepin	0	106	95
Imipramine	0	2345	2304
Other antidepressants:			
Mianserin	0	28	28
Trazodone	0	121	125
All drugs	**52 960**	**10 367**	**35 904**

Source: Stone et al. Risk of suicidality in clinical trials of antidepressants in adults: analysis of proprietary data submitted to US Food and Drug Administration. BMJ, 2009, Table 2 [271]. Used with permission of the publishers.

References Chapter 4

4. Borenstein M, Hedges LV, Higgins JP, Rothstein HR. Introduction to meta-analysis. 2009, Chichester, UK: John Wiley & Sons.

6. Higgins JPT, Green S, eds. Cochrane Handbook for Systematic Reviews of Interventions Version 5.1.0 [updated March 2011]. 2011, The Cochrane Collaboration. http://handbook.cochrane.org/.

8. U.S. Food and Drug Administration. Guidance for industry: Diabetes mellitus-evaluating cardiovascular risk in new antidiabetic therapies to treat Type 2 diabetes. 2008. http://www.fda.gov/downloads/Drugs/GuidanceComplianceRegulatoryInformation/Guidances/UCM071627.pdf.

9. Hammad TA, Laughren T, Racoosin J. Suicidality in pediatric patients treated with antidepressant drugs. Arch Gen Psychiatry, 2006, 63(3): 332-339.

10. Kim PW, Wu YT, Cooper C, Rochester G, Valappil T, Wang Y, Kornegay C, Nambiar S. Meta-analysis of a possible signal of increased mortality associated with cefepime use. Clin Infect Dis, 2010, 51(4): 381-389.

18. Moher D, Liberati A, Tetzlaff J, Altman DG, PRISMA Group. Preferred reporting items for systematic reviews and meta-analyses: the PRISMA statement. J Clin Epidemiol, 2009, 62(10): 1006-1012.

19. Stewart LA, Clarke M, Rovers M, Riley RD, Simmonds M, Stewart G, Tierney JF, Group P-ID. Preferred Reporting Items for Systematic Review and Meta-Analyses of individual participant data: the PRISMA-IPD Statement. JAMA, 2015, 313(16): 1657-1665.

20. Hutton B, Salanti G, Caldwell DM, Chaimani A, Schmid CH, Cameron C, Ioannidis JP, Straus S, Thorlund K, Jansen JP, Mulrow C, Catala-Lopez F, Gotzsche PC, Dickersin K, Boutron I, Altman DG, Moher D. The PRISMA extension statement for reporting of systematic reviews incorporating network meta-analyses of health care interventions: checklist and explanations. Ann Intern Med, 2015, 162(11): 777-784.

48. Hammad TA, Pinheiro SP, Neyarapally GA. Secondary use of randomized controlled trials to evaluate drug safety: a review of methodological considerations. Clin Trials, 2011, 8(5): 559-570.

49. Kalil AC. Is cefepime safe for clinical use? A Bayesian viewpoint. J Antimicrob Chemother, 2011, 66(6): 1207-1209.

59. CIOMS Working Group VI. Management of Safety Information from Clinical Trials. 2005, Geneva: Council for International Organizations of Medical Sciences.

105. Thompson SG, Higgins JP. How should meta-regression analyses be undertaken and interpreted? Stat Med, 2002, 21(11): 1559-1573.

126. Ioannidis JP, Lau J. Completeness of safety reporting in randomized trials: an evaluation of 7 medical areas. JAMA, 2001, 285(4): 437-443.

127. Pitrou I, Boutron I, Ahmad N, Ravaud P. Reporting of safety results in published reports of randomized controlled trials. Arch Intern Med, 2009, 169(19): 1756-1761.

132. Egger M, Davey Smith G, Schneider M, Minder C. Bias in meta-analysis detected by a simple, graphical test. BMJ, 1997, 315(7109): 629-634.

135. Yahav D, Paul M, Fraser A, Sarid N, Leibovici L. Efficacy and safety of cefepime: a systematic review and meta-analysis. Lancet Infect Dis, 2007, 7(5): 338-348.

139. Berlin JA, Santanna J, Schmid CH, Szczech LA, Feldman HI, Anti-Lymphocyte Antibody Induction Therapy Study G. Individual patient- versus group-level data meta-regressions for the investigation of treatment effect modifiers: ecological bias rears its ugly head. Stat Med, 2002, 21(3): 371-387.

140. Lambert PC, Sutton AJ, Abrams KR, Jones DR. A comparison of summary patient-level covariates in meta-regression with individual patient data meta-analysis. J Clin Epidemiol, 2002, 55(1): 86-94.

141. Schmid CH, Stark PC, Berlin JA, Landais P, Lau J. Meta-regression detected associations between heterogeneous treatment effects and study-level, but not patient-level, factors. J Clin Epidemiol, 2004, 57(7): 683-697.

163. Deeks JJ, Altman DG. Effect measure for meta-analysis of trials with binary outcomes. in Systematic reviews in health care: Meta-analysis in context, 2nd, M. Egger, G.D. Smith, and D.G. Altman, Editors. 2008, BMJ Publishing: London, UK.

164. Sutton AJ, Cooper NJ, Lambert PC, Jones DR, Abrams KR, Sweeting MJ. Meta-analysis of rare and adverse event data. Expert Rev Pharmacoecon Outcomes Res, 2002, 2(4): 367-379.

165. Deeks JJ. Issues in the selection of a summary statistic for meta-analysis of clinical trials with binary outcomes. Stat Med, 2002, 21(11): 1575-600.

166. Engels EA, Schmid CH, Terrin N, Olkin I, Lau J. Heterogeneity and statistical significance in meta-analysis: an empirical study of 125 meta-analyses. Stat Med, 2000, 19(13): 1707-1728.

167. Localio AR, Margolis DJ, Berlin JA. Relative risks and confidence intervals were easily computed indirectly from multivariable logistic regression. J Clin Epidemiol, 2007, 60: 874-882.

168. Grieve AP. The number needed to treat: a useful clinical measure or a case of the Emperor's new clothes? Pharm Stat, 2003, 2(2): 87-102.

169. Smeeth L, Haines A, Ebrahim S. Numbers needed to treat derived from meta-analyses-sometimes informative, usually misleading. BMJ, 1999, 318(7197): 1548-1551.

170. Parmar MK, Torri V, Stewart L. Extracting summary statistics to perform meta-analyses of the published literature for survival endpoints. Stat Med, 1998, 17(24): 2815-2834.

171. Williamson PR, Smith CT, Hutton JL, Marson AG. Aggregate data meta-analysis with time-to-event outcomes. Stat Med, 2002, 21(22): 3337-3351.

172. Moodie PF, Nelson NA, Koch GG. A non-parametric procedure for evaluating treatment effect in the meta-analysis of survival data. Stat Med, 2004, 23(7): 1075-1093.

173. Sutton AJ, Abrams KR, Jones DR, Jones DR, Sheldon TA, Song F. Methods for meta-analysis in medical research. 2000, Chichester, UK: J. Wiley.

174. Simmonds MC, Higgins JP, Stewart LA, Tierney JF, Clarke MJ, Thompson SG. Meta-analysis of individual patient data from randomized trials: a review of methods used in practice. Clin Trials, 2005, 2(3): 209-217.

175. Hedges LV, Olkin I. Statistical methods for meta-analysis. 1985, Orlando, FL: Academic Press.

176. Sweeting MJ, Sutton AJ, Lambert PC. Correction. Stat Med, 2006, 25: 2700.

177. Sweeting MJ, Sutton AJ, Lambert PC. What to add to nothing? Use and avoidance of continuity corrections in meta-analysis of sparse data. Stat Med, 2004, 23(9): 1351-1375.

178. Bennett MM, Crowe BJ, Price KL, Stamey JD, Seaman JW, Jr. Comparison of bayesian and frequentist meta-analytical approaches for analyzing time to event data. J Biopharm Stat, 2013, 23(1): 129-145.

179. Bradburn MJ, Deeks JJ, Berlin JA, Russell Localio A. Much ado about nothing: a comparison of the performance of meta-analytical methods with rare events. Stat Med, 2007, 26(1): 53-77.

180. Tian L, Cai T, Pfeffer MA, Piankov N, Cremieux PY, Wei LJ. Exact and efficient inference procedure for meta-analysis and its application to the analysis of independent 2 x 2 tables with all available data but without artificial continuity correction. Biostatistics, 2009, 10(2): 275-281.

181. Rucker G, Schwarzer G, Carpenter JR, Binder H, Schumacher M. Treatment-effect estimates adjusted for small-study effects via a limit meta-analysis. Biostatistics, 2011, 12(1): 122-142.

182. Yusuf S, Peto R, Lewis J, Collins R, Sleight P. Beta blockade during and after myocardial infarction: an overview of the randomized trials. Prog Cardiovasc Dis, 1985, 27(5): 335-71.

183. Greenland S, Salvan A. Bias in the one-step method for pooling study results. Stat Med, 1990, 9(3): 247-252.

184. Cai T, Parast L, Ryan L. Meta-analysis for rare events. Stat Med, 2010, 29(20): 2078-2089.

185. Firth D. Bias reduction of maximum likelihood estimates. Biometrika, 1993, 80(1): 27-38.

186. Heinze G, Schemper M. A solution to the problem of monotone likelihood in Cox regression. Biometrics, 2001, 57(1): 114-119.

187. The Handbook of Research Synthesis and Meta-analysis. 2nd ed. 2009, Russell Sage Foundation: New York, New York. 615.

188. Bailey KR. Inter-study differences: How should they influence the interpretation and analysis of results? Stat Med, 1987, 6(3): 351-358.

189. Peto R. Why do we need systematic overviews of randomized trials? Stat Med, 1987, 6(3): 233-244.

190. Poole C, Greenland S. Random-effects meta-analyses are not always conservative. Am J Epidemiol, 1999, 150(5): 469-475.

191. Berlin JA, Crowe BJ, Whalen E, Xia HA, Koro CE, Kuebler J. Meta-analysis of clinical trial safety data in a drug development program: answers to frequently asked questions. Clin Trials, 2013, 10(1): 20-31.

192. FDA. Reviewer Guidance: Conducting a Clinical Safety Review on a New Product Application and Preparing a Report on the Review. 2005. http://www.fda.gov/downloads/Drugs/GuidanceComplianceRegulatoryInformation/Guidances/ucm072974.pdf.

193. DerSimonian R, Laird N. Meta-analysis in clinical trials. Control Clin Trials, 1986, 7(3): 177-188.

194. Jackson D, Bowden J, Baker R. How does the DerSimonian and Laird procedure for random effects meta-analysis compare with its more efficient but harder to compute counterparts? J Stat Plan Inference, 2010, 140(4): 961-970.

195. Cornell JE, Mulrow CD, Localio R, Stack CB, Meibohm AR, Guallar E, Goodman SN. Random-effects meta-analysis of inconsistent effects: a time for change. Ann Intern Med, 2014, 160(4): 267-270.

196. IntHout J, Ioannidis JP, Borm GF. The Hartung-Knapp-Sidik-Jonkman method for random effects meta-analysis is straightforward and considerably outperforms the standard DerSimonian-Laird method. BMC Med Res Methodol, 2014, 14: 25.

197. Cochran W, Cox G. Experimental Designs. 2nd ed. 1992, New York: Wiley.

198. Higgins JP, Thompson SG. Quantifying heterogeneity in a meta-analysis. Stat Med, 2002, 21(11): 1539-1558.

199. Sutton AJ, Abrams KR. Bayesian methods in meta-analysis and evidence synthesis. Stat Methods Med Res, 2001, 10(4): 277-303.

200. Bayes TR. An essay towards solving a problem in the doctrine of chances. Philosophical transactions of the royal society of London, 1763: 370-418.

201. McGrayne SB. The Theory That Would Not Die: How Bayes' Rule Cracked The Enigma Code, Hunted Down Russian Submarines, & Emerged Triumphant from Two Centuries of Controversy. 2011, New Haven & London: Yale University Press.

202. Warn D, Thompson S, Spiegelhalter D. Bayesian random effects meta-analysis of trials with binary outcomes: methods for the absolute risk difference and relative risk scales. Stat Med, 2002, 21(11): 1601-1623.

203. Higgins JP, Thompson SG, Spiegelhalter DJ. A re-evaluation of random-effects meta-analysis. J R Stat Soc Ser A Stat Soc, 2009, 172(1): 137-159.

204. Lambert PC, Sutton AJ, Burton PR, Abrams KR, Jones DR. How vague is vague? A simulation study of the impact of the use of vague prior distributions in MCMC using WinBUGS. Stat Med, 2005, 24(15): 2401-2428.

205. Lee KJ, Thompson SG. Flexible parametric models for random-effects distributions. Stat Med, 2008, 27(3): 418-434.

206. Muthukumarana S, Tiwari RC. Meta-analysis using Dirichlet process. Stat Methods Med Res, 2012.

207. Mesgarpour B, Heidinger BH, Schwameis M, Kienbacher C, Walsh C, Schmitz S, Herkner H. Safety of off-label erythropoiesis stimulating agents in critically ill patients: a meta-analysis. Intensive Care Med, 2013, 39(11): 1896-1908.

208. Ohlssen D, Price KL, Xia HA, Hong H, Kerman J, Fu H, Quartey G, Heilmann CR, Ma H, Carlin BP. Guidance on the implementation and reporting of a drug safety Bayesian network meta-analysis. Pharm Stat, 2014, 13(1): 55-70.

209. Higgins JP, Spiegelhalter DJ. Being sceptical about meta-analyses: a Bayesian perspective on magnesium trials in myocardial infarction. Int J Epidemiol, 2002, 31(1): 96-104.

210. Askling J, Fahrbach K, Nordstrom B, Ross S, Schmid CH, Symmons D. Cancer risk with tumor necrosis factor alpha (TNF) inhibitors: meta-analysis of randomized controlled trials of adalimumab, etanercept, and infliximab using patient level data. Pharmacoepidemiol Drug Saf, 2011, 20(2): 119-130.

211. Kaizar EE, Greenhouse JB, Seltman H, Kelleher K. Do antidepressants cause suicidality in children? A Bayesian meta-analysis. Clin Trials, 2006, 3(2): 73-98.

212. Ibrahim JG, Chen MH, Xia HA, Liu T. Bayesian meta-experimental design: evaluating cardiovascular risk in new antidiabetic therapies to treat type 2 diabetes. Biometrics, 2012, 68(2): 578-586.

213. Hedges LV, Pigott TD. The power of statistical tests for moderators in meta-analysis. Psychol Methods, 2004, 9(4): 426-445.

214. Hedges LV, Pigott TD. The power of statistical tests in meta-analysis. Psychol Methods, 2001, 6(3): 203-217.

215. Hemminki E. Study of information submitted by drug companies to licensing authorities. BMJ, 1980, 280(6217): 833-836.

216. Easterbrook PJ, Berlin JA, Gopalan R, Matthews DR. Publication bias in clinical research. Lancet, 1991, 337(8746): 867-872.

217. Gotzsche PC. Reference bias in reports of drug trials. BMJ (Clin Res Ed), 1987, 295(6599): 654-656.

218. Gotzsche PC. Multiple publication of reports of drug trials. Eur J Clin Pharmacol, 1989, 36(5): 429-432.

219. Pocock SJ, Hughes MD, Lee RJ. Statistical problems in the reporting of clinical trials. A survey of three medical journals. N Engl J Med, 1987, 317(7): 426-432.

220. Tannock IF. False-positive results in clinical trials: multiple significance tests and the problem of unreported comparisons. J Natl Cancer Inst, 1996, 88(3-4): 206-207.

221. Heres S, Davis J, Maino K, Jetzinger E, Kissling W, Leucht S. Why olanzapine beats risperidone, risperidone beats quetiapine, and quetiapine beats olanzapine: an exploratory analysis of head-to-head comparison studies of second-generation antipsychotics. Am J Psychiatry, 2006, 163(2): 185-194.

222. Melander H, Ahlqvist-Rastad J, Meijer G, Beermann B. Evidence b(i)ased medicine—selective reporting from studies sponsored by pharmaceutical industry: review of studies in new drug applications. BMJ, 2003, 326(7400): 1171-1173.

223. Little RJ, Rubin DB. Statistical Analysis with Missing Data. 2002, Oxford, England: Wiley-Interscience.

224. National Institute for Health and Care Excellence (NICE). Guide to the Methods of Technology Appraisal. 2013. http://www.nice.org.uk/article/pmg9/chapter/Foreword.

225. National Institute for Health and Care Excellence (NICE). The guidelines manual. 2012. http://publications.nice.org.uk/the-guidelines-manual-pmg6.

226. Turner NL, Dias S, Ades AE, Welton NJ. A Bayesian framework to account for uncertainty due to missing binary outcome data in pairwise meta-analysis. Stat Med, 2015, 34(12): 2062-2080.

227. Higgins JP, White IR, Wood AM. Imputation methods for missing outcome data in meta-analysis of clinical trials. Clin Trials, 2008, 5(3): 225-239.

228. Biester K, Lange S. The multiplicity problem in systematic reviews. XIII Cochrane Colloquium. 2005, Melbourne, Australia. 153.

229. Baum ML, Anish DS, Chalmers TC, Sacks HS, Smith H, Jr., Fagerstrom RM. A survey of clinical trials of antibiotic prophylaxis in colon surgery: evidence against further use of no-treatment controls. N Engl J Med, 1981, 305(14): 795-799.

230. Lau J, Antman EM, Jimenez-Silva J, Kupelnick B, Mosteller F, Chalmers TC. Cumulative meta-analysis of therapeutic trials for myocardial infarction. N Engl J Med, 1992, 327(4): 248-254.

231. Flather MD, Farkouh ME, Pogue JM, Yusuf S. Strengths and limitations of meta-analysis: larger studies may be more reliable. Control Clin Trials, 1997, 18(6): 568-579; discussion 661-666.

232. Whitehead A. A prospectively planned cumulative meta-analysis applied to a series of concurrent clinical trials. Stat Med, 1997, 16(24): 2901-2913.

233. Pogue JM, Yusuf S. Cumulating evidence from randomized trials: utilizing sequential monitoring boundaries for cumulative meta-analysis. Control Clin Trials, 1997, 18(6): 580-93; discussion 661-666.

234. van der Tweel I, Bollen C. Sequential meta-analysis: an efficient decision-making tool. Clin Trials, 2010, 7(2): 136-146.

235. O'Brien PC, Fleming TR. A multiple testing procedure for clinical trials. Biometrics, 1979, 35(3): 549-556.

236. Lan KK, DeMets DL. Discrete sequential boundaries for clinical trials. Biometrika, 1983, 70(3): 659-663.

237. Kulinskaya E, Wood J. Trial sequential methods for meta-analysis. Res Synth Methods, 2014, 5(3): 212-220.

238. Imberger G, Wetterslev J, Gluud C. Trial sequential analysis has the potential to improve the reliability of conclusions in meta-analysis. Contemp Clin Trials, 2013, 36(1): 254-255.

239. Miladinovic B, Mhaskar R, Hozo I, Kumar A, Mahony H, Djulbegovic B. Optimal information size in trial sequential analysis of time-to-event outcomes reveals potentially inconclusive results because of the risk of random error. J Clin Epidemiol, 2013, 66(6): 654-659.

240. Higgins JP, Whitehead A, Simmonds M. Sequential methods for random-effects meta-analysis. Stat Med, 2011, 30(9): 903-921.

241. Thorlund K, Devereaux PJ, Wetterslev J, Guyatt G, Ioannidis JP, Thabane L, Gluud LL, Als-Nielsen B, Gluud C. Can trial sequential monitoring boundaries reduce spurious inferences from meta-analyses? Int J Epidemiol, 2009, 38(1): 276-286.

242. Brok J, Thorlund K, Gluud C, Wetterslev J. Trial sequential analysis reveals insufficient information size and potentially false positive results in many meta-analyses. J Clin Epidemiol, 2008, 61(8): 763-769.

243. Wetterslev J, Thorlund K, Brok J, Gluud C. Trial sequential analysis may establish when firm evidence is reached in cumulative meta-analysis. J Clin Epidemiol, 2008, 61(1): 64-75.

244. Jennison C, Turnbull BW. Meta-analyses and adaptive group sequential designs in the clinical development process. J Biopharm Stat, 2005, 15(4): 537-558.

245. Quan H, Ma Y, Zheng Y, Cho M, Lorenzato C, Hecquet C. Adaptive and repeated cumulative meta-analyses for safety signal detection during a new drug development process. Statistical Technical Report #54 (Sanofi), 2011, 54.

246. Lan KK, Hu M, Cappelleri JC. Applying the law of iterated logarithm to cumulative meta-analysis of a continuous endpoint. Statistica Sinica (Pfizer Inc.), 2003, 13: 1135-1145.

247. Hu M, Cappelleri JC, Lan KK. Applying the law of iterated logarithm to control type I error in cumulative meta-analysis of binary outcomes. Clin Trials, 2007, 4(4): 329-340.

248. Lau J, Schmid CH, Chalmers TC. Cumulative meta-analysis of clinical trials builds evidence for exemplary medical care. J Clin Epidemiol, 1995, 48(1): 45-57; discussion 59-60.

249. Chen MH, Ibrahim JG, Amy Xia HA, Liu T, Hennessey V. Bayesian sequential meta-analysis design in evaluating cardiovascular risk in a new antidiabetic drug development program. Stat Med, 2014, 33(9): 1600-1618.

250. Jeffreys H. An invariant form for the prior probability in estimation problems,. in Royal Statistical Society of London. 1946. London.

251. Bender R, Bunce C, Clarke M, Gates S, Lange S, Pace NL, Thorlund K. Attention should be given to multiplicity issues in systematic reviews. J Clin Epidemiol, 2008, 61(9): 857-865.

252. Thompson SG. Why sources of heterogeneity in meta-analysis should be investigated. BMJ, 1994, 309(6965): 1351-1355.

253. U.S. Food and Drug Administration. Guidance for industry non-inferiority clinical trials. US Department of Health and Human Services and US Food and Drug Administration, Washington, DC, 2010. http://download.bioon.com.cn/upload/201305/19233453_9245.pdf.

254. Deeks JJ, Altman DG, Bradburn MJ. Statistical methods for examining heterogeneity and combining results from several studies in meta-analysis. in Systematic Reviews in Health Care: Meta-analysis in context, 2nd edition, M. Egger, G.D. Smith, and D.G. Altman, Editors. 2001, BMJ Publishing Group: London.

255. Thompson SG, Sharp SJ. Explaining heterogeneity in meta-analysis: a comparison of methods. Stat Med, 1999, 18(20): 2693-2708.

256. Gagnier JJ, Moher D, Boon H, Bombardier C, Beyene J. An empirical study using permutation-based resampling in meta-regression. Syst Rev, 2012, 1: 18.

257. Morgenstern H. Uses of ecologic analysis in epidemiologic research. Am J Public Health, 1982, 72(12): 1336-1344.

258. Greenland S. Quantitative methods in the review of epidemiologic literature. Epidemiol Rev, 1987, 9: 1-30.

259. Oxman AD, Guyatt GH. A consumer's guide to subgroup analyses. Ann Intern Med, 1992, 116(1): 78-84.

260. Yusuf S, Wittes J, Probstfield J, Tyroler HA. Analysis and interpretation of treatment effects in subgroups of patients in randomized clinical trials. JAMA, 1991, 266(1): 93-98.

261. Rothwell PM. External validity of randomised controlled trials: "to whom do the results of this trial apply?" Lancet, 2005, 365(9453): 82-93.

262. Olkin I. Re: "A critical look at some popular meta-analytic methods". Am J Epidemiol, 1994, 140(3): 297-299; discussion 300-301.

263. Egger M, Smith GD, Sterne JA. Uses and abuses of meta-analysis. Clin Med, 2001, 1(6): 478-484.
264. Lewis S, Clarke M. Forest plots: trying to see the wood and the trees. BMJ, 2001, 322(7300): 1479-1480.
265. Stroup DF, Berlin JA, Morton SC, Olkin I, Williamson GD, Rennie D, Moher D, Becker BJ, Sipe TA, Thacker SB. Meta-analysis of observational studies in epidemiology: a proposal for reporting. Meta-analysis Of Observational Studies in Epidemiology (MOOSE) group. JAMA, 2000, 283(15): 2008-2012.
266. Liberati A, Altman DG, Tetzlaff J, Mulrow C, Gøtzsche PC, Ioannidis JP, Clarke M, Devereaux PJ, Kleijnen J, Moher D. The PRISMA statement for reporting systematic reviews and meta-analyses of studies that evaluate health care interventions: explanation and elaboration. PLoS Med, 2009, 6(7): e1000100.
267. Moher D, Shamseer L, Clarke M, Ghersi D, Liberati A, Petticrew M, Shekelle P, Stewart LA, PRISMA-P Group. Preferred reporting items for systematic review and meta-analysis protocols (PRISMA-P) 2015 statement. Syst Rev, 2015, 4: 1.
268. Shamseer L, Moher D, Clarke M, Ghersi D, Liberati A, Petticrew M, Shekelle P, Stewart LA, Group P-P. Preferred reporting items for systematic review and meta-analysis protocols (PRISMA-P) 2015: elaboration and explanation. BMJ, 2015, 349: g7647.
269. Zorzela L, Loke YK, Ioannidis JP, Golder S, Santaguida P, Altman DG, Moher D, Vohra S. PRISMA harms checklist: improving harms reporting in systematic reviews. BMJ, 2016, DOI: http://dx.doi.org/10.1136/bmj.i157. http://www.bmj.com/content/352/bmj.i157.
270. Hammad TA, Neyarapally GA, Pinheiro SP, Iyasu S, Rochester G, Dal Pan G. Reporting of meta-analyses of randomized controlled trials with a focus on drug safety: an empirical assessment. Clin Trials, 2013, 10(3): 389-397.
271. Stone M, Laughren T, Jones ML, Levenson M, Holland PC, Hughes A, Hammad TA, Temple R, Rochester G. Risk of suicidality in clinical trials of antidepressants in adults: analysis of proprietary data submitted to US Food and Drug Administration. BMJ, 2009, 339: b2880.
272. Lang T, Secic M. Considering "prior probabilities:" reporting Bayesian statistical analyses. in How to Report Statistics in Medicine: Annotated Guidelines for Authors, Editors, and Reviewers. 1997, American College of Physicians: Philadelphia. 231-235.
273. BaSiS Group. Bayesian Standards in Science: Standards for Reporting of Bayesian Analyses in the Scientific Literature. 2001. http://www.stat.cmu.edu/bayesworkshop/2001/BaSis.html.
274. Sung L, Hayden J, Greenberg ML, Koren G, Feldman BM, Tomlinson GA. Seven items were identified for inclusion when reporting a Bayesian analysis of a clinical study. J Clin Epidemiol, 2005, 58(3): 261-268.
275. Spiegelhalter DJ, Abrams KR, Myles JP. Bayesian approaches to clinical trials and health-care evaluation. 2004: Wiley. com.

CHAPTER 5.

INTERPRETATION OF RESULTS

5.1 Introduction

The purpose of this chapter is to describe a thought process for evaluating the findings of a meta-analysis beginning with first impressions, followed by a more thorough evaluation of the methodology, the fit with other evidence, and implications of the findings for potential subsequent regulatory actions. The chapter emphasizes that the results should be put into context with other available information on the benefits and risks of the product and that appropriate experts should be involved in the review. Section 5.2 discusses how the clinical importance of the meta-analysis will dictate the urgency with which it is necessary to communicate the results of the meta-analysis to relevant stakeholders (patients, regulatory agencies, marketing authorization holder). Section 5.3 provides a framework for evaluating the technical validity of the meta-analysis. Section 5.4 explains how to evaluate the reliability of the results and whether consistent conclusions can be drawn under a range of plausible assumptions. Section 5.5 explains how to integrate the results of a meta-analysis into the overall available information. It also explores how to interpret results from different sources to form an overall opinion on the benefit-risk balance of the product under review. This is further explored in section 5.6 which considers how a meta-analysis may have an impact on the labelling of a medicinal product and the need for further studies to be performed or additional risk minimization measures to be put in place by the marketing authorization holder. Finally, sections 5.7 and 5.8 discuss how the results of the meta-analysis should be reported and communicated. Section 5.8 includes recommendations on what information to include in the communication and also emphasizes that it is important that the information is communicated to the appropriate audience. It also stresses that it may be necessary to provide an interim communication after initial review of the meta-analysis that is followed later by more communications providing a more detailed review and more information on the implications of any change of use of the product as a consequence of the results of the meta-analysis.

Summary of main points:

▶ Meta-analysis may be performed before or after drug approval.

▶ The overall importance of the results should be assessed before diving into the details.

▶ Appropriate experts should be involved in the review.

▶ Results should be placed in context with other available information on the benefits and risks of the product.

The audience for a meta-analysis, regardless of when it is done, includes clinicians, statisticians, epidemiologists or other experts belonging to industry, academia, and regulators. If a meta-analysis becomes publicly available, the reader of a meta-analysis could in theory be anyone, but for the purposes of this chapter it is assumed to include at least the sponsor or the regulator unless otherwise stated. Assuming that the reviewer of a meta-analysis has patient responsibility (e.g. marketing authorization holder, regulator, or even prescriber) and wants to assess the results for further action needed to protect the safety of patients, the reviewer should consider some immediate questions prior to undertaking a more in-depth review:

▶ What is the potential clinical relevance of the meta-analysis? (see section 5.2)

▶ Has the meta-analysis been published in a journal with peer review? (Work that has not been peer-reviewed would require closer scrutiny. Conversely, publication in high-impact journals should not be taken as an automatic surrogate for the strength of the evidence. In effect, findings from published meta-analyses should be treated as "preliminary" evidence until these findings are verified with other streams of evidence.)

Once the urgency of further actions has been determined, an in-depth review of the meta-analysis should follow, addressing questions such as:

▶ What is the technical validity of the meta-analysis? See section 5.3.

▶ How robust are the results? See Chapter 3 and Chapter 4 and section 5.4.

▶ What is the strength of the totality of the evidence and is there existing supporting evidence for the findings? See section 5.5.

Review and assessment of the meta-analysis should be conducted with expertise from a wide range of specialties. Hence clinical, drug safety, and clinical pharmacology experts should be consulted to evaluate the clinical relevance of the findings, and experts in statistics and epidemiology should be consulted to evaluate the technical validity and methodological issues of the meta-analysis.

On the basis of these considerations the decision-making process can be initiated (see section 5.6) and ways of reporting and communication results should be discussed (see sections 5.7 and 5.8).

5.2 Potential clinical importance of the meta-analysis

Summary of main points:

▶ The likely public health impact influences the urgency of communicating the results, either by the marketing authorization holder or the relevant regulatory agency.

When a meta-analysis is published, the urgency of any actions to be taken by sponsors and/or by regulators needs to be evaluated by both parties in order to inform patients and health-care practitioners about potential risk in a timely manner. The reviewer should determine if the meta-analysis finds either a new, previously unknown risk, or an increase in frequency, specificity or severity of a known risk. If so, then this should be considered when the potential clinical importance and the plan for further assessment are considered, together with the decision-making process and the communication strategy.

At this stage, having not yet assessed the methodological quality of the meta-analysis, only the potential impact of the results can be considered.

The factors to consider should include:

▶ The nature and severity of the event: Is it plausible, preventable, treatable, reversible? Note: biological plausibility should be only a weak guidance, since lack of plausibility often means simply that we do not yet understand the causal mechanism, if any. As an example, consider diethylstilbestrol and the increase in risk of rare vaginal adenocarcinoma in female offspring exposed *in utero*, which could not be explained at the time [276].

▶ The extent of exposure of the population to the drug, the absolute risk (absolute numbers of patients potentially affected by the safety event) and the background incidence (if the effect size is reported as a ratio).

▶ Availability and suitability of licensed alternative treatments.

▶ The place of the new evidence in the totality of safety data about the product and its potential to substantially influence benefit/risk.

▶ Whether the evidence affects special populations such as children, older persons and pregnant women.

On the basis of these clinical considerations and the likely impact of available meta-analysis results on patients and physicians, the urgency and the suitable course of further actions can be decided.

5.3 Technical validity of the meta-analysis

Summary of main points:

▶ Check if the meta-analysis follows a pre-specified study protocol, and critically assess the methodological approach of the meta-analysis. More thorough methodological review is required if the meta-analysis was not published in a peer-reviewed journal, but publication by itself is not a guarantee of quality.

▶ Review the study characteristics and endpoint definitions of all studies included in the meta-analysis and assess potential sources of bias that might affect the meta-analysis results.

▶ Review the appropriateness and accuracy of the data extraction from the individual studies.

▶ Consider the level of multiplicity and the heterogeneity of study results. Assess medical plausibility, clinical relevance and consistency with other analyses when interpreting the meta-analysis results.

In this section the validity of the analysis performed is considered. Chapters 3 and 4 have discussed in detail appropriate methods for planning and conducting the analysis, and provide guidance on how to plan and to report meta-analyses in sections 3.1 and 4.10, respectively. These lists may be used as a reference to assess potential missing components or weaknesses in the analysis. In the case of meta-analyses submitted to regulatory authorities, there may be an opportunity to request additional information from the applicant. Based on the earlier material from this report, this section focuses on identifying major deficiencies in the meta-analysis that may have a substantive impact on the results and their interpretation and also on identifying when a meta-analysis should be considered to be reliable.

Consideration also has to be given to the accuracy of the data reported; where possible, individual study data should be compared to the source data to ensure accuracy and consistency of transcription.

5.3.1   Evaluating the plan for the meta-analysis

The first step should be to determine whether a meta-analysis protocol was prepared, whether this was done before or after data for the meta-analysis were assembled and analysis began, and whether the analysis presented is consistent with this protocol (see section 3.1 for the content of a protocol including the statistical analysis plan). Note that, in this context, a Program Safety Analysis Plan (PSAP; see Crowe et al. [60, 277] and Xia & Jiang [278] for more information on PSAPs) could be treated as the statistical analysis plan while a compound is in development. In the remainder of this chapter, our intention is to include the PSAP when we refer to a protocol or analysis plan.

Meta-analyses that are sufficiently planned before the analysis is done are always of higher credibility, as different types of biases are avoided or reduced. Ideally, the planning should be done before the results of the individual studies are known, if possible. If the final meta-analysis does not follow the original protocol, then the deviations from the protocol should be described and a reason for deviation should be given. Deviations should be relatively few, well explained and not driven by the results of the analyses.

The second step should be to assess critically the methodological approach taken in the meta-analysis protocol. Numerous principles are described in previous sections of this report, especially in Chapter 3 and Chapter 4. In general, a protocol should be reassuring regarding the potential multiplicity of analyses performed and the selection of data and methods that favour a particular result. Ideally the protocol focuses on a small number of potential research questions to be evaluated. If too many research questions are investigated with no ranking or order of assessment, even a planned meta-analysis may be difficult to evaluate. At a minimum, it may be possible to quantify the potential degree of selection among possible analysis choices, which is never possible for an unplanned analysis.

An extremely important topic in evaluating the meta-analysis protocol is the selection of studies to be included (see section 3.5). To assess whether the selection is appropriate the reader is recommended to consider section 3.5.1 where numerous examples of different situations are given. We highlight some key points here for reinforcement in the context of decision-making. Commonly, in the case of an investigational drug, the developer of the drug has access to and can include all data available, or some relevant subset, such as all controlled trials. This is an ideal situation, but in other cases those performing the analysis may have to resort to literature searches, and be limited by the data that have been published. It is important to assess whether the search strategy is comprehensive: was an attempt made to identify and collect data from unpublished studies? Are the selected studies appropriate for the proposed evaluation? For example, if an effect is expected to emerge only over an extended period, should studies of short duration be included? Similar questions may be asked regarding inclusion of studies with multiple indications, and perhaps the inclusion of several different drugs with similar mechanism of action. All of these are subjective evaluations. As noted in sections 3.2 and 3.5, there are many possible situations in which meta-analysis may be applied, so the reviewer must consider both whether the choice of studies was pre-specified and whether this choice seems appropriate.

The plan should clearly identify the outcomes to be evaluated (see sections 3.3 and 3.4). Since safety endpoints are often not the primary outcome measures in clinical trials, they may, for instance, be collected only as AEs through open-ended (non-specific) questioning of the patient. However, it is important to evaluate whether the data available for the meta-analysis are likely to be accurate and complete. Is the information of interest likely to have been elicited from the patient and recorded in the study database? (Note that we are not necessarily advocating that every possible event be elicited. For example, a psychiatrist might be unlikely to ask a patient about weight gain unless the study protocol specifically requires that information. However, knowing whether the specific event was elicited or not can help assess the completeness of the information.) Is there any differential ascertainment between the groups? Is the information on AEs recorded in a consistent way from study to study? If the data were obtained from publications, and a given study reports no events, is it because there were no events, because the events were collected but not reported, or because the events were never elicited? Is the outcome one that has a subjective component? If so, was there any attempt to adjudicate or in some other way ensure consistency? (We note that for some endpoints, such as all-cause mortality, adjudication is probably not needed, although completeness of ascertainment still needs consideration.) Have individual participant data or summary data been used for the meta-analysis?

One example with a standard, predefined search strategy was the set of meta-analyses performed to evaluate risk of suicidality (now referred to as suicidal ideation and behaviour) in patients treated with antidepressants. A summary of these meta-analyses is provided in Appendix 1. For the original meta-analysis, the data were provided to the US FDA by the sponsors of the included trials and a standard, predefined, search strategy was used within each trial to identify potential cases. Each case was then adjudicated by a blinded independent reader. This type of process may provide more consistent and reliable data than would be possible from the trial source data only.

The most thorough meta-analyses will include a pre-specified plan for subgroup analyses and analyses evaluating the sensitivity of the primary analyses (see section 4.9). Although appropriate subgroup analysis and interaction testing is encouraged, it should be noted that an excess of subgroup analyses or focus of the study results on subgroups rather than the overall population raises concerns about multiplicity. The fact that subgroups are specified in a plan does not eliminate the problem that examining many subgroups creates an increased chance of false positive results (because of multiplicity), or false negatives (particularly if formal adjustment for multiplicity is used). There can be several problems. First, multiplicity adjustment could mask treatment effects within subgroups, considering that subgroups are often inherently underpowered.) Second, true differences in treatment effects between subgroups may also fail to be detected because of multiplicity adjustment. Nonetheless, greater credibility should be given to subgroup results when that specific subgroup was identified for particular attention in the analysis plan (e.g. young adults in the example on antidepressants).

Section 4.2 has discussed the issue of zero-event studies. The analysis plan should address both whether such studies are captured in the studies included for analysis and consideration of appropriate analysis methods. (Zero event studies were frequent in the analyses of antidepressant drugs, and rosiglitazone (Appendix 4) and additional analyses were performed as suggested in section 4.2, although not reported in detail in the papers). If the results of a specific study have triggered the meta-analysis, the analysis plan should specify an approach to assessing the contribution of this study to the overall result. Although it is logical to follow up such a finding, there is a risk that including the hypothesis-generating study may lead to an overestimate of the effect.

Even very thorough meta-analyses including all available data may still be underpowered. It is therefore important to consider *a priori* what size of effect might be clinically relevant and consistent with the hypothesized mechanism (see section 4.5). In addition, even if the meta-analysis is technically valid, results of a single trial should have been replicated by other trials to avoid drawing wrong conclusions [279]. Examining the CI will give useful information about the potential range of effect sizes, although as with P values the nominal confidence may be overstated due to multiplicity.

5.3.2 Potential for obtaining an incorrect answer (including potential for bias and applicability of findings to populations of interest)

The previous section has covered a number of points about the planning phase that also reflect on the quality of the meta-analysis itself. In this context, quality refers to the extent to which the meta-analysis can provide the basis upon which to draw a valid conclusion. Even a technically well-conducted meta-analysis is limited by the adequacy of the available studies and their potential for bias. A more thorough discussion of potential sources of bias in individual studies can be found in section 3.8. Where the studies are identified from the literature, unpublished data will be missing, leading to a risk of publication bias (discussed in section 4.6.1). There may be other reasons for failing to retrieve particular studies (e.g. failing to include studies in languages other than English. The completeness and consistency of endpoint definitions is harder to check, especially if access to the individual participant data in the original databases was not available and the meta-analysis is based only on summary results.

In addition to considering potential biases, how well the results of the meta-analysis can be applied to the population of interest should also be evaluated. In particular:

▶ Is the population of each study relevant to the meta-analysis objective; how do the age range, comorbidities and concomitant treatments compare to a "real life" population?

▶ When was the study conducted and have there been any changes in medical practice that may affect its relevance?

Funnel plots [132, 133] can be used to detect different types of bias, as discussed in section 3.8.4. Briefly, in analyses based on published studies, publication bias can result from the failure to include unpublished data combined with the preference of academic journals to publish studies on the basis of the direction or statistical significance of results and the failure of authors to submit studies based on the nature of the findings [216]. Studies with positive results are often more likely to be referenced in subsequent publications, which may affect the studies selected if the search strategy is not comprehensive [217]. Study results can also influence the likelihood that the study will be reported in multiple publications, and so care must be taken to ensure that duplicate data are not included in the meta-analysis [6, section 10.1, 218]. Bias may also result from selective reporting of analyses (e.g. subgroups) or of outcomes (e.g. changing the primary or secondary outcomes from what was specified in the original clinical trial protocol) within published trials [65, 66] or changes in plan. These may be analyses and outcomes that were planned in the study protocol but not considered relevant for publication on the basis of the results, or they may be unplanned analyses and outcomes that have been defined post hoc and were considered relevant for publication, also on the basis of the results. It is therefore important not to rely solely on the published data, but also to check the published information vs. the originally-planned analyses and outcomes if the study protocols are accessible.

Finally, there is always a dilemma about the scope of studies to be included in the meta-analysis. As noted above (section 3.1), one analysis should correspond to minimal selection decisions – i.e. using as much data as possible from the original trials and imposing as few opinions of the meta-analysts as possible.

Only then does it become obvious what effect these opinions have. However, another view is that the aim should be to run a meta-analysis with as many unbiased trials as possible, even if this is only a subset of all trials. This may be pre-specified by restricting the primary analysis to a set of studies with stricter filters on the reliability of their results. Sensitivity analyses should have been performed to determine if there are any potential limitations in the conclusions drawn from the results of the meta-analysis.

5.3.3 Multiplicity

Evaluation of safety problems is often associated with multiple analyses and multiple testing. Within the context of exploratory safety analyses, multiplicity is associated with an inflated rate of false positive findings and the need for control of type I error. Meta-analyses evaluating safety concerns seldom include clinical trials where the safety variable under study was part of the confirmatory strategy of the study, mostly because such primary studies are rarely conducted. In addition, they often do not form part of a pre-planned development plan of the drug. In situations such as these, results are fundamentally of an exploratory nature.

When interpreting results of a meta-analysis, two different scenarios might be differentiated with regard to the interpretation of P values. First, the performed meta-analysis can be an explicitly planned part of a drug development programme. In that case, the consequences of multiple testing have been discussed previously and a multiplicity adjustment or hierarchy for testing endpoints would have been pre-specified. This does not mean that all potential multiplicity has been removed, or that all associations rendered non-significant by any adjustment for multiplicity are untrue, but the expectation is that a logical approach to reducing multiplicity has been carefully considered and that nominal P values need to be interpreted in this context. The second scenario relates to meta-analyses that are not planned parts of the development programme and that have been conducted outside this programme by a sponsor or by an external party. In this case, issues of multiplicity have in general not been considered a priori and no adjustment for multiplicity has been performed. There is also greater potential for such analyses to be data-driven, which leads to other multiplicity issues. A meta-analysis of a single specific concern, based on a well-thought-out hypothesis, perhaps suggested by a plausible mechanism of action, can be very convincing. Yet the same data arrived at as part of a "data dredging" or data-driven operation (e.g. in response to a published article that raises a specific safety concern) can be difficult to interpret. This is not to argue against meta-analysis as part of routine safety monitoring, but only to emphasize the difficulties in interpreting statistical significance.

When evaluating adverse effects observed in a meta-analysis, discussion of P values has limitations, as the observation of substantial differences will raise concerns depending on the seriousness and severity of the outcome, irrespective of the observed P value. Thus, absence of statistical significance does not necessarily rule out a safety concern. The interpretation of safety data needs to be performed in the context that less evidence may be needed to take action on a possible harm, as compared to assessments of efficacy, where efficacy is only considered to be established when conclusive evidence is available. While from a statistical point of view, there might be issues related to post hoc analyses and multiplicity, in the context of safety concerns and taking into account the overall body of data at hand, data might be considered sufficient for regulatory actions despite limitations with regard to frequentist significance testing.

Conversely, statistical significance does not necessarily establish existence of a safety concern. Results of a meta-analysis need to be evaluated taking into account the magnitude of the observed effect estimates, CIs and P values (and noting that both CIs and P values are subject to multiplicity). Consideration should be given to limitations of purely dichotomous interpretations of P values. In the context of lack of multiplicity adjustment for multiple testing, a possible increase in the probability of false positive findings has to be weighed against the importance of not missing a safety concern.

In evaluating the level of multiplicity within the meta-analysis, the number of endpoints, the clinical importance of those endpoints, the number of subgroups and the consistency of the results should be considered. As an illustration, we take the example of suicidality evaluation in adults treated with antidepressants [271] (see Appendix 1). As illustrated in Figure 5.1, the overall results of the meta-analysis suggested modest evidence of a beneficial effect in reducing suicidality. However, in the subgroup of youngest patients (<25 years old) there is a substantial increase in risk, and using a statistical test of interaction there is a suggestion that this group is not consistent with the remaining age groups (P = 0.004 for interaction). In this meta-analysis the age group <25 years had been identified prospectively as the subgroup of greatest interest. Based on previous data in children evaluated using the same methodology, there was also evidence of a similar increase in risk. The existing evidence and prior hypotheses regarding a potential age effect therefore lend credibility to the specific risk in young adults. A similar subgroup finding in different circumstances may well have been dismissed as likely to be due to random chance.

Figure 5.1 Odds of suicidality (ideation or worse) for active drug relative to placebo by age in adults with psychiatric disorders

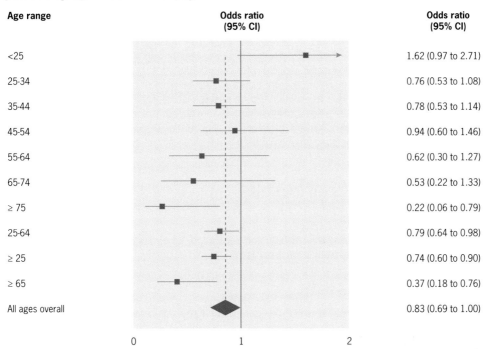

Age range	Odds ratio (95% CI)
<25	1.62 (0.97 to 2.71)
25-34	0.76 (0.53 to 1.08)
35-44	0.78 (0.53 to 1.14)
45-54	0.94 (0.60 to 1.46)
55-64	0.62 (0.30 to 1.27)
65-74	0.53 (0.22 to 1.33)
≥ 75	0.22 (0.06 to 0.79)
25-64	0.79 (0.64 to 0.98)
≥ 25	0.74 (0.60 to 0.90)
≥ 65	0.37 (0.18 to 0.76)
All ages overall	0.83 (0.69 to 1.00)

Source: Stone et al. Risk of suicidality in clinical trials of antidepressants in adults: analysis of proprietary data submitted to US Food and Drug Administration. BMJ, 2009, Figure 2 [271]. Used with permission of the publishers.

5.3.4 Heterogeneity of treatment effects

Sections 4.3.4 and 4.8 discuss the causes and evaluation of heterogeneity. The presence of statistical evidence for heterogeneity of treatment effects among the included studies does not necessarily affect the interpretation of results. It is important to evaluate the clinical relevance of the heterogeneity. Differences that are quantitative (i.e. reflecting differences in magnitude of the effect, but not direction) rather than qualitative (i.e. differences in the direction of the effect across studies) probably do not affect the interpretation of the overall results. However, qualitative differences require further investigation. In some situations, when there is a specific study-design or population factor of interest (e.g. more severe vs. less severe illness), it may be appropriate to perform a specific interaction test of that factor, rather than rely on a global test of heterogeneity. This is because there could be variability in treatment effects across levels of a specific factor, even in the absence of an overall significant test for heterogeneity.

As an example, earlier in the chapter (Figure 5.1) the results of the evaluation of suicidality in patients receiving antidepressants were discussed and shown in a forest plot. If a meta-analysis were performed that included all studies, both adult and paediatric, a clear heterogeneity between the paediatric studies (showing a harmful effect) and the adult studies (showing a generally beneficial effect in most adults) would be observed.

To some extent, heterogeneity may also reflect the choice of scale for the analysis. Most meta-analyses are based on relative measures of effect (e.g. RR, ORs) that represent a treatment effect proportional to the underlying risk. This allows for inclusion of data with a wide range of baseline risks, but it should be kept in mind that treatment differences assessed on a relative scale are not constant on an absolute scale if the baseline risk differs. In some cases, it may be more appropriate to use an absolute measure of risk (risk difference, or RD) when the baseline risk and the RD are relatively consistent between studies. This distinction may be important, as for example in the case of aspirin which decreases the risk of ischemic events (MI or ischemic stroke) but also (by virtue of the same mechanism of action) increases the risk of haemorrhagic stroke. In a population that has a high baseline (untreated) risk of ischemic events, a 25% relative reduction could lead to a substantial reduction in absolute risk. In a population with a low baseline (untreated) risk of ischemic events, the 25% relative reduction would produce a smaller absolute reduction in risk. However, if the baseline (untreated) risk of haemorrhagic stroke does not vary between these two populations, because some risk factors for bleeding differ from the risk factors for ischemic events, the absolute increase in risk due to aspirin could be relatively constant across the populations. Thus, the absolute reduction in ischemic risk, compared with the absolute increase in haemorrhagic risk, could represent a very different trade-off in the high ischemic risk population than in the low-risk population and, as such, will have an impact on the evaluation of the benefit-risk balance in these two patient populations.

5.4   Robustness of results

Summary of main points:

▶ Considerations for evaluating the reliability and consistency of results are discussed, including the limitations of assumptions made in the analysis.

▶ Design factors such as disease status, background therapy, dose regimen, and study size and duration may have an impact on the findings.

▶ Plausibility and relevance of the clinical outcome as a measure of the risk being assessed needs to be evaluated.

▶ The nature and multiplicity of analysis decisions and strength of evidence (P value, results of sensitivity analyses) also have an impact on the credibility of results.

In this section, how to evaluate the reliability and consistency of the results considering any limitations of assumptions made in the analysis will be discussed. The main concerns can be divided into three areas: a) those concerns related to the design of the included studies; b) those related to the clinical relevance of the endpoints; and c) those related to the analysis itself. To some extent, each concern can be examined by sensitivity or subgroup analysis, as described in sections 4.8 and 4.9. For each sensitivity or subgroup analysis, those analyses predefined in an analysis plan should be given greater credibility than those that are not predefined. However, it should be kept in mind that, even when they were pre-specified, having planned an excessive number of subgroup analyses does not avoid the issue of multiplicity. Nevertheless, not all planned analysis decisions are the correct ones, so the reviewer must make his or her own assessment of each analysis decision. Generally, if the reviewer believes the approach is valid (regardless of whether he/she would have chosen the same approach), then the primary analysis and the overall study results should be given greater credibility, and the extent to which sensitivity or subgroup analyses show contradictory evidence would need to be substantial before moving away from this default position. Alternatively, if the reviewer believes that a particular analysis decision is clearly inappropriate, corresponding sensitivity or subgroup analyses may be given greater credibility. If the initial decision to include all drugs in a particular chemical class, for example, appears reasonable because of a common hypothesized mechanism of action, then subgroup analysis for each drug would be given less weight. In many situations, the opinions of more than one reviewer will be helpful, as different reviewers bring different expertise to the review.

5.4.1 Concerns related to the design of the included studies

As noted in section 5.3.2, study design factors may be important to consider when evaluating a meta-analysis. Specific design factors of interest would include (but not be limited to) the following:

▶ Differences in dose regimen (or drug in the case of analyses based on a class of drugs), background therapy, comorbidity and indication.

▶ Differences in study duration (both between studies and possibly between different treatment groups with the same study), particularly if an AE is believed, based on clinical knowledge, to occur soon after exposure begins (e.g. immediate allergic reactions), or only after prolonged exposure or follow-up (e.g. cancer).

▶ Differences in population studied.

▶ Is the control or comparator group always the same; is there a placebo or active control, and what are the background therapies?

▶ Outcome: was the outcome measure within each study planned or unplanned, were there consistent definitions across studies or not, was there adjudication of endpoints (if needed), and were there any possible ascertainment differences between the treatment arms?

▶ Blinding: when outcomes are subjective this is very important, but less so in the case of hard endpoints such as mortality.

▶ Completeness of the data, extent of dropout/loss to follow-up (attrition).

▶ Unit of analysis issues: did the level of analysis align with the level at which randomization occurred? Were adjustments for so-called "design effects" applied in the analysis?

As an example, each of these factors was considered as part of the evaluation of suicidality risk for paediatric patients treated with antidepressants [9] (see Appendix 1 for details). Data for nine drugs were included; although these represented several different classes of drugs, the mechanisms hypothesized for an effect on suicidality have typically been related to a general antidepressant effect rather than a specific pharmacological process. The original trigger for this meta-analysis was a report on paroxetine, so some consideration should be given to the data for this drug separately, but otherwise it seems reasonable to form an initial hypothesis in which the same effect is shared by all drugs. The provided subgroup analysis shows that, although no events were reported for two of the drugs, the remaining drugs all show a trend for increased risk, and two of the drugs have a relative risk greater than that for paroxetine. Analysis of the data excluding paroxetine also confirmed the overall finding. Results are also provided for the subgroup of medications, selective serotonin reuptake inhibitors (SSRIs), to which paroxetine belongs.

Continuing the example, three-quarters of the studies were of patients with major depression. The remaining studies were in other psychiatric conditions, including several in indications not approved for any of the drugs other than paroxetine. Nevertheless an *a priori* decision to include these other indications seems reasonable, assuming the patients could be expected to be at increased risk of suicidality and to also have some depressive symptoms. Results show that the estimated treatment effect is similar whether based on all trials or only on those in major depression. The control group in all cases is placebo. There is an absence of information on the trial durations, which would need to be addressed, but typically the duration of placebo-controlled trials in depression is short due to ethical concerns and therefore there is unlikely to be any large variation in the duration of the included trials. The absence of long-term controlled studies would preclude evaluation of changes in risk over time.

Section 3.5 has discussed some particular concerns based on the size of the included studies. There is a possibility that small published trials may exaggerate the effect size when compared to larger trials, possibly due to publication bias. Figure 5.2 presents an example in which meta-analysis of different treatments for osteoarthritis showed ($P < 0.05$) evidence of such small study effects in 4 out of 13 meta-analyses studied [280]. In Figure 5.2, the estimates and CIs represent the difference in average treatment effect between a meta-analysis of small studies (those with fewer than 100 patients per group) and a meta-analysis of larger studies. Where subgroup analyses show evidence of such an effect, then the reviewer must consider whether the entirety of the overall effect could be attributed to bias, or whether the remaining data provide enough evidence of an effect, albeit smaller than originally estimated. This may present a difficult decision, even if the data suggest that small trials are associated with larger effect sizes. In the absence of a conclusive explanation as to how this bias arose, it may be necessary in the interest of protecting patient safety, to take a position that a risk may still exist even if the quantification of this risk is put into doubt. Some methods have been proposed to adjust for small trial biases and sensitivity analyses based on these methods will be helpful in assessing the potential magnitude of bias [181, 281].

Each "intervention" is a meta-analysis of a pain-related outcome. The "difference in effect sizes" shown is the difference in pain score between a meta-analysis of small (fewer than 100 patients per arm) trials and a meta-analysis of large (at least 100 patients per arm) trials for the given intervention. The "P value for interaction" is based on a test of whether the effect size for pain scores for the meta-analysis of small trials differs from the effect size for pain scores from the meta-analysis of large studies of the same intervention. The average difference in effect sizes between large and small trials across the 13 included meta-analyses was −0.21 (95% CI: −0.34 to −0.08, P = 0.001), suggesting that the small trials on average showed more beneficial effects.

Figure 5.2 Small study effects in meta-analyses of osteoarthritis

Intervention	Difference in effect sizes (95% CI)	Difference in effect sizes (95% CI)	P value for interaction
Acupuncture		-0.63 (-1.10 to -0,17)	0.007
Aquatic exercise		-0.10 (-0.63 to 0.43)	0.71
Balneotherapy		-0.85 (-1.84 to 0.15)	0.10
Chondroitin		-0.66 (-1.06 to -0.26)	0.001
Diacerein		-0.15 (-0.37 to 0.07)	0.18
Exercise		-0.12 (-0.28 to 0.05)	0.15
Glucosamine		-0.78 (-1.26 to -0.30)	0.001
Opioids		-0.12 (-0.29 to 0.05)	0.18
Oral NSAIDs		-0.19 (-0.49 to 0.12)	0.23
Paracetamol		0.28 (-0.26 to 0.82)	0.31
Self management		0.05 (-0.13 to 0.23)	0.57
Topical NSAIDs		-0.10 (-0.32 to 0.13)	0.40
Viscosupplementation		-0.35 (-0.63 to -0.06)	0.018
Overall (τ^2 = 0.03, P=0.005)		-0.21 (-0.34 to -0.08)	

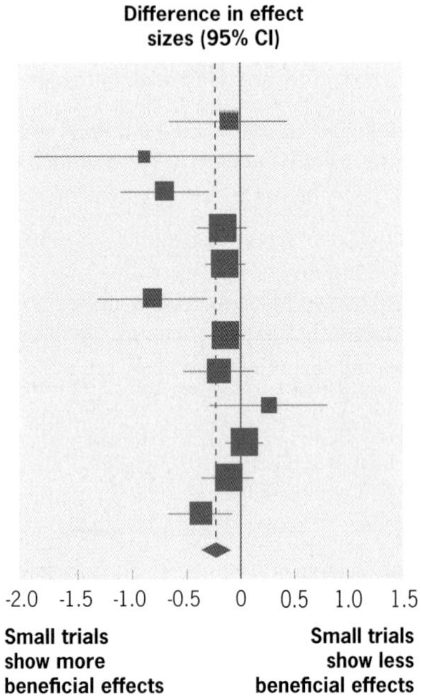

-2.0 -1.5 -1.0 -0.5 0 0.5 1.0 1.5

Small trials show more beneficial effects   **Small trials show less beneficial effects**

Source: Nüesch et al. Small study effects in meta-analyses of osteoarthritis trials: meta-epidemiological study. BMJ, 2010, 341, Figure 1 [280]. Used with permission of the publishers.

5.4.2 Concerns related to the clinical relevance of the endpoints

The focus now turns to consideration of clinical relevance. These factors may be of a more subjective nature and harder to address with additional analysis than those discussed previously. Given the duration of the clinical trials included, is it plausible that there is a causal relationship between the studied treatment and the outcome? For example, studies of short duration would be unlikely to detect a causal effect in a slow-growing tumour or in atherosclerotic progression but could detect events such as thrombosis or acute renal failure.

The time at which the trials were conducted should be considered. Trials conducted many years in the past may not reflect modern practice. This may be related to the drug under study (e.g. dosing regimens of chemotherapy agents and treatment combinations may change substantially over time) or to the background therapies that have evolved over time. If possible, the specific factors that have changed should be investigated directly but in some cases, due either to lack of access to individual data or the multiplicity of factors, time can be a useful surrogate. Evidence of increasing or decreasing risk over time should be weighed as part of the overall benefit-risk assessment. However, careful interpretation is warranted. The fact that calendar year of publication can sometimes be a useful surrogate might also mean that time is also strongly associated with more than one study-level factor, so disentangling the source of variability can be challenging.

The clinical relevance of the endpoint also has to be considered, including evaluation of the individual components in cases in which the endpoint is a composite with components that may represent different levels of severity (e.g. minor vs. major bleeding). Even when the outcomes have clearly-understood long-term consequences, it may still be complex to evaluate outcomes that have widely varying rates across different subpopulations.

A more complex evaluation is required for the example of suicidality, which has previously been discussed. Completed or attempted suicide represents a clear outcome, but in the meta-analysis of paediatric trials there were no such events, and among adults there were only a few such events. Therefore much of the analysis relies on the interpretation of events of suicidal ideation. Although it seems logical that increased ideation should be associated with increased risk of an actual suicide attempt, research on this topic is unclear and is complicated by the difficulty in eliciting accurate information on the patient's mental status. There are also wide variations in the rates of suicide with age and sex. In particular, the groups identified as having increased risk of suicidality (children and young adults), have the lowest rates of completed suicide. This is an example in which the actual risk to the patient is very poorly defined but, since ideation is a necessary step to an action, it seems prudent (though this is a judgement) to consider that some risk of completed suicide may exist.

5.4.3 Concerns related to the analysis itself

Finally, with regard to robustness, some topics related to the analysis itself are relevant. Some deviations from the analysis plan are to be expected as part of logical follow-up of the initial findings. These deviations should be relatively few and should be well-explained and not driven by the findings of individual studies or of initial meta-analyses. Changing the definition or importance of outcomes after seeing the results can lead to biased and misleading conclusions [282]. However, there could be situations in which an unexpected finding, or an outlier, could give rise to a reasonable hypothesis that was not considered in the planning of the analysis. For example, suppose all attempts fail to explain heterogeneity of findings, using pre-specified characteristics of studies or populations. Closer examination of the observed data could generate hypotheses for future consideration or modelling. One might find that studies with larger effect sizes were all conducted prior to a certain calendar time, which in turn corresponds to the time at which a particular aspect of a treatment regimen (e.g. concomitant therapy) was changed. Because the hypothesis was generated by observing the data, a formal hypothesis test would be invalid, but that hypothesis might be tested in a related clinical area.

The robustness of the result is reflected to some extent in the P value for the primary analysis. If the P value is very small (say <0.001), then it is less likely that the various sensitivity or subgroup analyses will seriously challenge the finding that some increased risk is present. This point needs to be tempered, however, by considering both the point estimate of the treatment effect and its variance. A low P value could be robust to sensitivity analyses in the presence of a small effect size and very small variance, but if the sensitivity analyses do not address the underlying source of bias, the reassurance provided by apparent robustness could be misleading. Similarly, multiplicity issues will also be of less concern because adjustments for multiplicity would not change the conclusions. Cumulative meta-analysis raises its own concerns (see section 4.7). In the absence of any widely accepted approach to dealing with multiplicity issues, the reviewer should at least be aware that it is not uncommon for findings to be reversed [283].

Lack of consistency between the subgroups also requires investigation to ensure that this is not a sign of some more fundamental problem with the analysis (see the discussion in section 5.3.4 regarding the choice of scale for analysis and its relation to heterogeneity of effect). Sections 4.8.1 and 4.8.3 have described many of the issues related to subgroup analyses. Generally, results from a single subgroup of a meta-analysis should be given low credibility, although we should recognize that such a result could be true. If multiplicity has not already been accounted for, the reviewer may wish to apply informal corrections to P values according to the number of subgroups examined. An exception would be situations in which a particular subgroup was of *a priori* concern based on some prior evidence. For example, in the investigation of suicidality in adults treated with antidepressants (Appendix 1, [271] and Figure 5.1) there was already evidence of an effect in children, and the analysis plan identified young adults as the primary subgroup of interest. Thus, although the primary analysis hypothesis was that a risk existed for all adults, the finding of an interaction with age, and increased risk in young adults was credible and consistent with other data.

Section 4.3 discusses the choice of fixed-effect vs. random-effects models. In many cases, a random-effects analysis will lead to a slightly greater (less significant) P value, and wider CIs compared with a fixed-effect analysis, so such differences should be expected if a sensitivity analysis is performed. Larger differences between the analyses (e.g. dramatically different point estimates of effect) suggest that the different weighting applied to the studies is having an important effect. As discussed in section 4.3.1, a careful examination of the results in small studies should be performed before concluding which analysis is more credible.

5.5   Integration and interpretation of evidence

Summary of main points:

▶ The clinical and medical relevance of the safety concern, and the impact for patients, need to be considered for interpretation. This includes impact on symptoms and quality or quantity of life and also depends on predictability, preventability and reversibility of the reaction or event.

▶ The importance of the meta-analysis for the safety concern under study needs to be determined by taking into account the limitations of the study as well as its external validity. This is mainly determined by the quality of the meta-analysis itself and by how far the results may apply to populations exposed to the product in medical practice.

▶ Results of the meta-analysis have to be integrated in the overall context of other available information, which may encompass non-clinical data, data from other clinical and observational studies, and results from other analyses, such as from spontaneous reporting. Each source of evidence has to be assessed individually for its appropriateness, quality and validity and has to be integrated conceptually into the overall available data on the safety concern, after careful evaluation with regard to validity and generalizability. Strengths of different sources of evidence relating to data in the efficacy context do not necessarily match with the strengths of evidence in the safety context.

Evaluation of safety concerns arising from meta-analyses and other sources encompasses various aspects that are not limited to the evaluation of data included in the meta-analysis itself. As for any safety concern, the clinical and medical relevance of the safety aspects observed have to be taken into account. Section 5.5.1 covers these aspects in more detail in addition to the high-level information provided in section 5.2. Evaluation of aspects of the meta-analysis itself includes the meta-analysis' validity, robustness, limitations and external validity. Most of these aspects have been discussed in detail in sections 5.3 and 5.4. However, some high-level aspects of these issues are discussed here as they are important for weighing the evidence generated in the meta-analysis in the context of the totality and weight of all evidence available. Section 5.5.2 gives an overview of aspects that are important for weighing the evidence of a meta-analysis. For reaching an overall conclusion on the adverse effect under evaluation, different sources of evidence relating to a safety concern will have to be assessed and will lead to an overall interpretation of the safety concern. Section 5.5.3 gives an overview of how different sources of evidence might be incorporated into an overall assessment. The overall available data on a safety concern would then be evaluated taking into account available data on benefit, leading to a benefit-risk assessment (see section 5.8.2).

5.5.1 Clinical and medical relevance of the safety concern and patient impact

As noted, at a high level in section 5.2, which addresses the preliminary assessment one would do, prior to understanding the methods used in the meta-analysis, the clinical importance of a safety concern will depend on the impact of the AE on patients' symptoms, quality or quantity of life (e.g. mild gastrointestinal symptoms would be of less significance than a major gastrointestinal bleeding event, or permanent neurological damage or unexpected death). However, the acceptance of the risk of occurrence of any adverse effects of a drug will also depend on the expected benefits and the severity and morbidity of the treated condition, which forms part of a benefit-risk assessment (see also section 5.8.2).

Further aspects of clinical relevance include predictability, preventability and reversibility of the reaction or event [284]. It should be noted that not all of these aspects might be addressed in a meta-analysis and that other data might have to be taken into account for further clarification of these points.

Predictability of events relates to their risk of occurrence and, more specifically, to how well occurrence of a reaction might be anticipated, how possible risk factors might influence the risk of occurrence, and the extent to which individual or subgroup characteristics might modify an adverse effect of treatment. For example, it may be that the increase in risk of a specific AE is limited to certain subgroups of patients. This appears to be the case in the suicidality example, in which only younger patients demonstrate the increased risk associated with antidepressants. Knowledge about predictability is closely related to its preventability, to the extent that knowledge about possible risk factors could permit targeted risk mitigation activities, which are discussed below.

One way to frame the question of predictability is that, when evaluating a safety concern, the absolute as well as the relative risk (including the precision of the respective estimates) of the event needs to be taken into account. While relative risk estimates comparing the risk under treatment to a comparison group might be high, the absolute risk might be very low, thereby indicating that a small number of treated patients are affected by the AE. The public health importance of the frequency of occurrence of an AE will in general be related to an absolute scale, although a meta-analysis may analyse and report results on a relative scale. Therefore, absolute risks will always need to be considered in addition to relative risks. However, it has to be considered that transformation of relative risks into absolute risks might be subject to certain limitations, such as dependency on time-scale. In addition, absolute risks will be dependent on baseline risks that may differ in different populations and subgroups.

A second aspect of predictability is that evidence for potential differential effects with regard to subgroups of special populations needs to be taken into account when evaluating the safety concern. By differential effects, we mean here that the relative effect of treatment on the risk of the AE is different in different subgroups. Relevant data might arise from meta-analyses evaluating different populations (e.g. the meta-analysis leading to evaluation of the safety concern), but evidence might also relate to other sources of observational or other data. Consideration should be given to patient characteristics that might be relevant to the risk under evaluation. For instance, age, disease severity, patients with hepatic or renal impairment, other comorbidities, genetic polymorphisms or characteristics such as pregnancy or lactation might be factors that could potentiate or mitigate the risk of occurrence associated with treatment.

Preventability is related to the potential for risk reduction. There might be instances where risk reduction, and therefore a certain degree of preventability of an adverse effect, might be achieved only through restriction of access – such as by excluding certain patient populations at higher intrinsic absolute risk of an adverse effect (e.g. those with several risk factors) from treatment. For example, suppose a drug is found to double the risk of an AE. A patient who has a 1% risk of that event even in the absence of treatment would have his or her risk increased to 2%. A patient with a 10% intrinsic risk would have that risk doubled to 20%, a much bigger absolute increase. Such considerations relating to patient populations might also be addressed in meta-analyses, and appropriate analyses might provide useful information to determine populations at higher or lower risk of AEs. In other situations, prevention might be achieved by modifying the method of intake or route of administration. Such aspects might be related to pharmacological or biological aspects and would therefore only rarely be addressed by a meta-analysis of clinical trials, unless those pharmacological or biological aspects are also captured in the trials, thus permitting appropriate subgroup analyses.

Aspects of reversibility of adverse effect could potentially be addressed by meta-analyses, but typically would relate to pharmacological and clinical aspects that would be based on clinical or preclinical data apart from meta-analyses. As with preventability, in order to be addressed analytically, data related to these factors would need to have been captured during the clinical trials and could then define appropriate additional analyses. Alternatively, it might be possible to perform combined analyses of the preclinical data or the early-phase clinical data. Such analyses go beyond the scope of this report.

An important factor to consider is the extent of utilization of the product in the general population and in special populations, implying the need for an assessment of whether utilization takes place in populations at higher or lower risk. The size of the population using a medicinal product will clearly determine the actual number of potentially affected patients and will be important to assessment of the public health impact.

The medical importance of an AE also depends on the availability of other therapeutic options that might themselves be associated with other AEs or that might have a less well characterized safety profile, leading to higher uncertainty with regard to the probability of occurrence of adverse effects. In some circumstances, these AEs might be more severe than the risk identified by the meta-analysis and might affect a larger number of patients than the actual risk under evaluation. A possible effect of discontinuation of treatment might have serious or only limited consequences. Discontinuing a drug with urgent medical need might have worse consequences than the adverse effect under discussion. For example, discontinuation of substitutive treatment (e.g. insulin in insulin-dependent diabetes) might simply not be possible in most clinical situations. Discontinuing effective anticancer treatment would need careful evaluation of the individual benefit-risk context. However, discontinuation of a drug used for weight reduction where other non-pharmacological interventions are available might not have the same serious consequences as discontinuation of drugs in the previously mentioned settings.

The risk under evaluation might also depend on dose and route of treatment, so the duration of treatment relative to the period of risk needs to be considered as well. These points might also have been addressed in the meta-analysis and, similarly, the time- or dose-dependency of effects might have been subject to subgroup analyses or meta-regression. However, caution would be necessary if the meta-analysis included non-approved and higher-than-approved dosages. Analyses of dose-dependency might inform the plausibility of a signal, but not all aspects of these analyses might be relevant for clinical practice if this relates to higher-than-approved doses. Aspects of time-dependency need careful evaluation in meta-analyses since the length of follow-up and the period at risk might be different (e.g. occurrence of cancer, if induced or promoted by a drug, might be detected only several years after treatment and might not always or even typically be included in the follow-up time of trials included in a meta-analysis). Another caveat with regard to examining dose-dependency relates to trials using flexible dosing regimens. As mentioned in section 3.5.1, caution should be exercised because, in this scenario, an observed association between drug exposure and a given AE might be inaccurate due to the dynamics that allow participants to move between various levels of dosing in a manner that might be dependent on experiencing the AE [48].

The importance of a safety concern might be further characterized by the existing awareness and novelty of an AE. From a regulatory perspective, this might be determined by whether the risk of the AE is included in the product information or whether it has already been addressed in a risk management plan or in periodic safety update reports/periodic benefit risk evaluation reports.

These considerations also form part of a benefit-risk evaluation (see also section 5.8.2).

5.5.2 Weighing the importance of the meta-analysis for the safety concern under study

An interpretation of the results of a meta-analysis needs to take into account the limitations of the analysis as well as the extent of external validity of the study. Sections 5.3 and 5.4 have discussed aspects of internal validity and robustness in detail. These include:

- whether the meta-analysis was properly planned;

- the quality of study data from the clinical trials included in the meta-analysis;

- heterogeneity of the findings across studies and across subgroups within studies; and

- duration of follow-up relative to the expected time course of the AE (if known).

Critical additional points for assessing the importance and relevance of the meta-analysis with regard to the safety concern under evaluation will be presented here.

The importance of a meta-analysis could depend on the appropriateness of the choice of comparator. Trials in the analysis might include a placebo or an active treatment comparison. A treatment might increase risk relative to placebo but, if an active comparator was used and that comparator also increases risk of the same AE, no difference between the experimental treatment and the active comparator might be detected. Combination of placebo groups and groups of patients receiving active treatment might therefore be problematic, but separate meta-analyses with the different comparators would be very informative. This would have to be based on a thorough evaluation of available data, taking into account problems related to multiple testing and not just basing conclusions on a dichotomous interpretation of *P* values.

Relevance of the meta-analysis will depend on the representativeness of the population included in the meta-analysis. Populations exposed in medical practice might differ substantially from those included in clinical studies. In clinical practice, risk for AEs, or susceptibility to the increase in risk caused by exposure, could differ from what was observed in the clinical trials, as a result of the inclusion or exclusion criteria in the trials leading to selection of patients. For example, metformin is contraindicated in patients with severe renal impairment because of their higher risk of experiencing lactic acidosis.

Clinical trials evaluating metformin in comparison to other drugs are therefore likely to exclude patients with severe renal impairment. An absence of risk of lactic acidosis in meta-analyses of these clinical trials might therefore not be indicative of the non-existence of this risk in patients with severe renal impairment. A signal could be missed either because the relative risk due to treatment varies between populations, or because the low baseline risk in the trial population did not provide enough statistical power (enough events of interest) to detect the signal.

5.5.3 Context of the safety concern

Apart from the data relating to the meta-analysis itself, the interpretation of a safety concern needs to take into account the context of the safety concern and the data from the meta-analysis have to be integrated in the overall context of other available information.

This may encompass non-clinical data, data from single interventional or clinical studies, observational studies, results of other meta-analyses or data from spontaneous reporting systems. It should be noted that, in general, no superiority of one data source over another can be assumed since different sources will have different strengths in different situations. Each source of evidence has to be assessed individually and has to be integrated conceptually into the overall available data on the signal after careful evaluation with regard to validity and generalizability. As this report focuses on meta-analysis, only criteria for the evaluation of results from meta-analysis are presented in detail. However, the concepts outlined in section 5.5.2 will, in principle, apply to evaluation of each source of evidence, although some adaptation will be necessary depending on the nature of data evaluated (e.g. observational data might undergo a thorough evaluation of problems related to unmeasured confounding, while nonclinical data might be subject to an evaluation of whether the conduct of studies has been performed according to relevant guidelines).

Such an evaluation of each source of evidence may include consideration of the pharmacological and biological plausibility of the signal under discussion (and available evidence for this) and the question as to whether a mechanism of action might exist that could explain the observed effect. However, in many instances, a biological mechanism might be explored or discussed only after a safety concern has been observed or established. In other words, the signal from a meta-analysis (or other sources) could lead to experiments aimed at discovering the biological mechanism, rather than the other way around. Other points to consider would be the temporal association(s) observed and its plausibility with regard to the AE.

A discussion of the overall available evidence relating to a safety signal would also need to differentiate between prior available evidence on the safety problem and evidence that might arise after a signal has been detected. For example, the results of a meta-analysis, or of a published epidemiological study, might influence the generation of later data (e.g. induced spontaneous reporting or a prompted hypothesis concerning pharmacological theories on the effect under study). In the USA, in particular, early findings might generate litigation and high media publicity, which in turn could generate a spike in spontaneous reporting.

When evaluating other sources of data, one should consider that the strengths of different sources of evidence relating to data in the efficacy context do not necessarily match with the strengths of evidence in the safety context. The strength of the evidence is determined by the quality of the data or study in terms of appropriateness of methods to address the question under evaluation. It is also determined by the internal and external validity of the study and its generalizability, rather than by the design itself. Data that will be regarded as high quality and evidence for efficacy purposes might have important shortcomings with regard to specific safety outcomes (e.g. if the sample size was not high enough to evaluate the occurrence of rare events or if populations with specific risk factors were excluded from the studies). Whereas efficacy would in general be established by compelling pivotal randomized controlled trials, these trials might be insufficient to address certain safety aspects. For evaluation of these aspects, further studies would have to be conducted. For example, information on fluoroquinolones and tendon disorders or gadolinium-containing contrast agents and nephrogenic systemic fibrosis primarily emerged from spontaneous case reporting and clinical trials were not able to evaluate these associations.

While evidence from clinical trial data and from well-designed meta-analyses on safety issues will, in general, be regarded as high strength of evidence, in some specific circumstances observational data or other sources of data could be regarded as being of higher relevance and could thus be highly important for the overall evaluation. This might be the case, for example, when the safety event under study is very rare or populations are affected that might not be easily included in clinical trials (e.g. safety events such as venous thromboembolism, retinal detachment or safety issues relating to newborns or pregnant women). Absence of data from clinical trials might in those cases be related to the limitations of the randomized trial design with regard to the safety question at hand, rather than to the non-existence of this event (e.g. a too-limited sample size for appropriate ascertainment of a specific safety event.

In such cases, other sources of data, such as observational data, might represent high strength of evidence if methods are appropriate and robust against bias and confounding. All sources of data and of evidence have to be assessed for their appropriateness, quality and validity and the results of the meta-analysis have to be interpreted in the context of the overall data. In some cases, data other than a meta-analysis of randomized trials might be of greater importance or may play a more important role in the overall interpretation based on the above considerations.

5.6 Impact on use of medicinal products

Summary of main points:

▸ Meta-analysis findings may have an impact on many regulatory activities concerning a drug, including changes to professional labelling, risk minimization plans and requests for further studies.

▸ Meta-analysis findings may be considered as new safety information.

> ▶ Drug sponsors should notify the relevant regulatory bodies when they become aware of a new meta-analysis with clinically significant findings pertaining to one of their drugs.

> ▶ Meta-analysis findings should be interpreted in conjunction with the total information available about the drug.

> ▶ Resolution of uncertainty about the conduct or the findings of the meta-analysis might require additional information, data or further studies.

When a meta-analysis provides evidence of a clinically important and previously unknown effect of a treatment, this may require changes to the way the product is used and may possibly result in requests for further information. Different parties may be called upon to make decisions, including regulators, drug sponsors, health-care providers, patients, and health-care systems and payers. The focus of this section will be on regulators and drug sponsors, who have direct roles in the authorization of approved uses of the drug. The primary attention will be on the decision process specific to meta-analysis findings; however, attention is also given to the process for safety findings in general that are relevant to meta-analysis findings.

A safety finding from a meta-analysis, like a finding from other sources, may ultimately result in a range of regulatory actions, including additions of warnings in the approved label, changes in the approved use in the label, restrictions on the access to the drug, enhanced pharmacovigilance, educational efforts and additional studies. Changes may also be required to the risk management plan for the product. Both regulators and drug sponsors may have internal advisory bodies to consider safety issues and enforce or suggest specific actions. In certain cases, based on the context of the meta-analysis, public advisory groups may be convened to make recommendations on actions.

There are other elements of the decision-making process in the regulatory context related to meta-analysis. The findings of a meta-analysis may be considered new safety information requiring certain actions of the drug sponsor, including changes to the drug label and the conduct of additional studies. These actions may be initiated by the sponsor but may also be requested or required by a regulator. Hence, an essential prerequisite is early and full communication between the sponsor and regulators. In Europe, such communication is covered by Volume VI of Good Pharmacovigilance Practice (see section VI.C.2.2.6), [285] which introduces the concept of an "emerging safety issue", which is a class of safety problems that should be notified to regulators at the earliest opportunity. It is expected that drug sponsors inform regulators of the existence of any publicly available meta-analysis or meta-analysis submitted to another regulatory body that may have bearing on the safety of a drug.

In general, any safety findings are part of a collection of information and knowledge of the drug based on pharmacology, preclinical studies, pivotal randomized clinical trials, dedicated safety trials, spontaneous reporting, registries, observational studies and knowledge of the drug class. The information and knowledge are continually evolving. The necessary inputs for the decision process are: (1) assessment of the validity of the design and conduct of the meta-analysis, and (2) assessment of the context of the meta-analysis findings. These topics are the subject of previous chapters and previous sections of this chapter and include: the severity of the safety outcome, the estimated effect of the drug on the outcome, the number of people potentially at risk, the overall benefit-risk profile of the drug, and the degree to which the findings represent potentially new knowledge on the safety profile of the drug. A team with the necessary expertise, including clinical experts on the drug and statistical experts on meta-analysis, should be used for assessment of the validity of the meta-analysis. To assess the context of the meta-analysis, additional experts may be required, including experts on drug utilization and subject matter experts for specific studies that have bearing on the risk and benefits of the drug.

The assessments of the validity and the context of the meta-analysis jointly affect the decision process. Even a meta-analysis with important limitations may result in specific decisions given the assessment of the context. For example, for a newly marketed drug with limited information on its use in clinical practice, a meta-analysis with large uncertainty may warrant safety communications or enhanced pharmacovigilance.

The uncertainty of the meta-analysis findings can be reduced, enabling more effective decisions, by identifying and addressing the limitations of the meta-analysis. The resources devoted to resolving the uncertainty of the meta-analysis should take into account the assessment of the context of the meta-analysis and the likelihood that the resolution would change the decision. The regulators and drug sponsors may address some of the uncertainty in the meta-analysis by requesting additional information from the meta-analysis authors or by conducting additional analysis based on information presented in the study report, as well as additional information that might have not been publicly available. If the protocol and analysis plan were not made publicly available, the regulators and drug sponsor should request these from the study authors. They may also request additional summaries and analyses from the study authors that address uncertainty or methodological concerns.

For a meta-analysis based on limited, publicly available data, regulators can request that the drug sponsor conduct a more thorough meta-analysis. The drug sponsor probably has access to patient-level trial data and possibly trial results that have not been published (although it might be hoped that all newer trials would be published). With patient-level data, outcome definitions used in the original trials might be improved in terms of validity and consistency if the requisite data are available. In addition, differential exposure patterns, time patterns of the events, and subgroups can be explored for consistency or for the identification of groups at greater risk. The drug sponsor may be able to identify additional trials, including trials that they have sponsored, contributed to, or of which they are otherwise aware.

Regulators may choose to expand a meta-analysis of a single drug to a review of the relevant drug class. This can be done to understand the safety outcome for the entire class or to increase the available data on the safety issue. Because of confidentiality and propriety concerns, a regulatory body may be the only party capable of producing a thorough class-wide meta-analysis, although in some instances a neutral party, other than the regulator or the sponsor, might be engaged, as was the case in the meta-analysis by Askling et al. [210].

5.7 Reporting of results

Summary of main points:

▶ The method used to select trials and patients is an important part of the report.

▶ When reporting results of a meta-analysis, absolute effect sizes should be presented in addition to relative effect sizes.

A checklist of items that would be expected to appear in the report of a meta-analysis is provided in Table 4.1 (presented in section 4.10.2).

A flow diagram (such as Figure 4.3 in section 4.10.2) illustrates well how the final set of trials and patients has been selected for the meta-analysis.

Part of each meta-analysis report should be a presentation of the meta-analysis population and an overview of the number of patients per drug. (Table 4.2 is an example of such a presentation in section 4.10.2.)

A forest plot has been discussed earlier in this report as being a suitable tool for comparing the effect sizes of the safety endpoint of interest among all trials included into the meta-analysis. In addition, it summarizes nicely the single and meta-analysis results of the effect measure, the variability within and among trials and the weight each trial contributes to the meta-analysis. Note that consideration also should be given to the potential for selective reporting of endpoints, or subgroup or other analyses, within individual studies. Refer also to section 4.10.1 and section 4.6 for further information and guidance on forest plots and other issues related to missing data.

The majority of meta-analyses present the effect size as a relative risk or OR. However, for interpretation of risk from a public health perspective, the absolute effect size should also be presented, together with some measure of how the effect of treatment on absolute risk may vary according to the baseline risk of the various patient populations that the drug would be used in. Depending on the availability of data and the willingness to assume constancy of the effect size across trials, one might conduct the analysis using more than one metric (e.g. ORs and RDs), or conduct the analysis on one scale (e.g. OR) and then convert the summary measure to another metric. Localio et al. propose a method for converting from OR to other metrics [167]. Perception of risk can be influenced by the way in which it is presented and presentation as on an absolute scale is more correctly interpreted by both patients and medical professionals [286]. For example, warfarin used to treat atrial fibrillation reduces the risk of ischemic stroke by 60% but increases the risk of haemorrhagic stroke by 200%. Presented in this way this may suggest that use of warfarin is harmful. However, if it is understood that the underlying risk of haemorrhagic stroke is much lower than that of ischemic stroke, then we may understand that the absolute risk of ischemic stroke is reduced by 3% and the absolute risk of haemorrhagic stroke increased by 1%.

5.8 Communication of results

Summary of main points:

▶ The process of communication of safety findings from meta-analyses is closely related to other processes of risk communication. Guidance documents and reports are available on this topic (e.g. [287]).

▶ Risk communication is a process in which all stakeholders have to be aware of their responsibilities, with the safety of patients as paramount. There is a need for clear and accurate reporting of safety findings that should also take into account transparency on the interpretation of findings and uncertainties related to the results.

▶ Information needs to reach the right audience at the right time to allow implementation of timely and appropriate actions. Different levels of detail and explanation may be necessary depending on the specific concerns of different audiences.

▶ The process of interpretation of safety issues may involve different steps of assessment, which may lead to different scenarios of communication and may involve early communication. Early communication, before completion of a full review, is important in situations where interim measures need to be implemented or patients currently on the medication should stop taking it as soon as possible. In cases where early communication is provided, it is important to note that further important information that emerges from subsequent analyses of information must be communicated in a timely manner.

▶ When communicating results of a meta-analysis, absolute effect sizes should be presented in addition to relative effect sizes.

Apart from factual reporting of results, appropriate ways of communicating the results from a meta-analysis should be taken into consideration. The process of communication of safety findings from meta-analyses is closely related to other processes of risk communication and there are guidance documents and reports available on this topic (e.g. *Dialogue in pharmacovigilance* by the Uppsala Monitoring Centre, and the European Medicine Agency's *Good Pharmacovigilance Module XV – Safety Communication*) [287-289]. A thorough discussion on the whole topic of risk communication is beyond the scope of this report. This section will therefore focus on discussion of some important principles of risk communication that are relevant to meta-analyses.

The communication of safety findings involves different stakeholders such as regulatory agencies, biopharmaceutical sponsors, journalists, researchers, physicians and patients. Although each of these may have different perspectives and different interests with regard to the safety findings at hand, risk communication is also a process where all stakeholders have to be aware of their responsibilities, with the safety of patients as paramount. This responsibility calls for a clear and accurate reporting of safety findings that should also take into account transparency in the interpretation of findings and uncertainties related to the results. Moreover, any constraints need to be declared, such as prior agreement with other parties that may affect the complete reporting of the information when the information is first known. Such situations include not being the actual owner of the outcome data or situations in which the provision of full information is embargoed.

For the relevant stakeholder who is involved in communicating the safety findings, the information needs to reach the right audience at the right time to allow implementation of timely and appropriate actions. It has to be noted that different levels of detail and explanation may be necessary depending on different audiences that have to be informed (e.g. health-care professionals, members of the public or media), while transparency should be ensured independently of the level of detail to be provided.

5.8.1   Communication at different stages of analyses

The process of interpretation of safety issues may involve different steps of assessment, which may lead to different scenarios of communication, depending on the stage of assessment. On the basis of the safety issue at hand, and in the light of transparency, plans should be made for the different stages of communication of the assessment results, so that timely information is provided.

Early communication, before completion of a full review, is important in situations where interim measures need to be implemented or patients currently on the medication should stop taking it as soon as possible. We note, however, that there is clearly a level of judgement involved in determining whether or not the current situation falls into this category. If an interim result is presented, the interim nature of the information should be mentioned up front, but it should also be noted that it is being provided in the interest of maintaining full transparency of the situation and that further updates will be provided when they are available. Even though a final analysis has yet to be made, review of the data to that point in time has shown safety issues and physicians may need to re-evaluate the choice of therapy in their patients. (Again, different individuals might have a different threshold for what constitutes a safety issue that needs to be communicated.)

The risks involved should be clearly spelt out and relevant guidance for both physicians and patients should be provided to prevent potential confusion. Note that problems can arise from inappropriately hasty communication of interim results. In some situations, an interim analysis might show an increased risk of a particular harm that might lead patients to stop treatment, possibly without consulting with their health-care providers. The risks associated with discontinuation of treatment might also be substantial, so a dialogue between the patient and the health-care provider is crucial. There is also the potential for patients to be channelled from one drug to others in the same class which might end up, after full investigation, to be associated with the same risk [290]. Importantly, if the interim results are not supported by subsequent analyses, any consequences of discontinuation would have been avoidable, but only in hindsight. Thus, in cases where early communication is provided, it is important to note that further important information that emerges from subsequent analyses of information must be communicated to both physicians and patients in a timely fashion.

5.8.2   Benefit-risk evaluation incorporating information from the meta-analysis

Regulators are increasingly focusing on highlighting and maintaining a positive benefit-risk balance for new interventions. Recent discussions aim at a more transparent decision process as to whether benefits outweigh risks or not, how to deal with uncertainties and how to manage risks. It is worth noting that a meta-analysis represents a piece of information from the overall data relevant to a benefit-risk evaluation. A meta-analysis may evaluate one single safety issue on the basis of a selection of all data collected in different trial settings. However, the process of benefit-risk evaluation often goes beyond evaluation of a single meta-analysis, thereby taking into account other sources of data and evaluating both risks and benefits. Therefore, if results from a meta-analysis reveal or confirm a safety finding, information on all important risks of the affected medicinal product should be presented in the context of the main benefits of the medicine. Available information on the seriousness and severity of the safety finding need to be provided, together with information on the frequency of the safety finding, relevant risk factors, time to onset and reversibility (and time to resolution) of adverse reactions.

Results of the benefit-risk evaluation should be communicated by clearly indicating uncertainties and limitations with regard to benefits and risks, possible risk minimization, and the weights and importance of these issues. A summary-level meta-analysis on a well-ascertained outcome may be sufficient to rule out a given level of risk and could support a favourable benefit-risk profile of a drug. In contrast, a previously unidentified, potential safety signal that would substantially affect the benefit-risk profile of a drug may necessitate large efforts in resolving the uncertainties of the meta-analysis. One should address whether, and to what extent, the results of the meta-analysis influenced the evaluation of the benefit-risk balance and whether there is any change regarding this assessment compared to earlier benefit-risk assessments. Important emerging information based on the meta-analysis results should be indicated, as well as how the benefit-risk balance under different conditions of use are thereby affected.

5.8.3   Guidance arising from the meta-analysis and the benefit-risk evaluation

In addition to presenting an evaluation of the results and putting it into the perspective of the benefit-risk profile of the medicinal product, any recommendation to health-care professionals and patients on how to deal with the safety concern should be clearly stated. Specific guidance should be provided to stakeholders (e.g. hospitals, clinic patients or general physicians) on whether treatment with, or usage of, the concerned product should be continued and whether the treatment needs to be changed. Risks of alternative treatments and risks related to the avoidance or cessation of the concerned drug should be considered and clearly communicated. Guidance may also be required on how to safely switch to alternative treatments.

If applicable, information on any proposed change to the product information should also be provided. Literature references and additional sources of more detailed information should be indicated, where available.

5.8.4   Interaction of authors/journal editors and regulatory agencies

Although manuscripts submitted to journals are clearly confidential prior to publication, authors and journal editors should be aware of their responsibilities for adequate and balanced dissemination of data, especially with regard to drug safety findings. To ensure timely evaluation of safety data and appropriate communication processes, both authors and journal editors may want to consider informing regulatory agencies prior to publication of drug safety findings. Findings may be submitted prior to publication under confidentiality agreements. Care should be taken to ensure that the regulatory agencies understand when reports coming from both a journal and the authors are referring to the same finding.

5.9   Concluding remarks

The results of a meta-analysis of relevant safety data require careful interpretation to initiate appropriate actions to protect the safety of patients while under drug treatment.

This chapter has shown how complex and time-consuming the interpretation process might be. However, a structured approach (see section 5.1) guides the reviewer of a meta-analysis through the steps for the synthesis of evidence, the decision-making process and, finally, proper communication.

Depending on the stage of the life cycle of the drug when the meta-analysis is performed and on the potential clinical relevance, the urgency of further actions and the complexity of the interpretation will vary greatly.

References Chapter 5

6. Higgins JPT, Green S, eds. Cochrane Handbook for Systematic Reviews of Interventions Version 5.1.0 [updated March 2011]. 2011, The Cochrane Collaboration. http://handbook.cochrane.org/.

9. Hammad TA, Laughren T, Racoosin J. Suicidality in pediatric patients treated with antidepressant drugs. Arch Gen Psychiatry, 2006, 63(3): 332-339.

48. Hammad TA, Pinheiro SP, Neyarapally GA. Secondary use of randomized controlled trials to evaluate drug safety: a review of methodological considerations. Clin Trials, 2011, 8(5): 559-570.

60. Crowe BJ, Xia HA, Berlin JA, Watson DJ, Shi H, Lin SL, Kuebler J, Schriver RC, Santanello NC, Rochester G, Porter JB, Oster M, Mehrotra DV, Li Z, King EC, Harpur ES, Hall DB. Recommendations for safety planning, data collection, evaluation and reporting during drug, biologic and vaccine development: a report of the safety planning, evaluation, and reporting team. Clin Trials, 2009, 6(5): 430-440.

65. Al-Marzouki S, Roberts I, Evans S, Marshall T. Selective reporting in clinical trials: analysis of trial protocols accepted by The Lancet. Lancet, 2008, 372(9634): 201.

66. Dwan K, Gamble C, Williamson PR, Kirkham JJ, Reporting Bias G. Systematic review of the empirical evidence of study publication bias and outcome reporting bias - an updated review. PLoS One, 2013, 8(7): e66844.

132. Egger M, Davey Smith G, Schneider M, Minder C. Bias in meta-analysis detected by a simple, graphical test. BMJ, 1997, 315(7109): 629-634.

133. Sterne JA, Harbord RM. Funnel plots in meta-analysis. Stata Journal, 2004, 4: 127-141.

167. Localio AR, Margolis DJ, Berlin JA. Relative risks and confidence intervals were easily computed indirectly from multivariable logistic regression. J Clin Epidemiol, 2007, 60: 874-882.

181. Rucker G, Schwarzer G, Carpenter JR, Binder H, Schumacher M. Treatment-effect estimates adjusted for small-study effects via a limit meta-analysis. Biostatistics, 2011, 12(1): 122-142.

210. Askling J, Fahrbach K, Nordstrom B, Ross S, Schmid CH, Symmons D. Cancer risk with tumor necrosis factor alpha (TNF) inhibitors: meta-analysis of randomized controlled trials of adalimumab, etanercept, and infliximab using patient level data. Pharmacoepidemiol Drug Saf, 2011, 20(2): 119-130.

216. Easterbrook PJ, Berlin JA, Gopalan R, Matthews DR. Publication bias in clinical research. Lancet, 1991, 337(8746): 867-872.

217. Gotzsche PC. Reference bias in reports of drug trials. BMJ (Clin Res Ed), 1987, 295(6599): 654-656.

218. Gotzsche PC. Multiple publication of reports of drug trials. Eur J Clin Pharmacol, 1989, 36(5): 429-432.

271. Stone M, Laughren T, Jones ML, Levenson M, Holland PC, Hughes A, Hammad TA, Temple R, Rochester G. Risk of suicidality in clinical trials of antidepressants in adults: analysis of proprietary data submitted to US Food and Drug Administration. BMJ, 2009, 339: b2880.

276. Herbst AL, Ulfelder H, Poskanzer DC. Adenocarcinoma of the vagina. Association of maternal stilbestrol therapy with tumor appearance in young women. N Engl J Med, 1971, 284(15): 878-881.

277. Crowe B, Xia HA, Nilsson ME, Shahin S, Wang WV, Jiang Q. The program safety analysis plan: An implementation guide. in Quantitative evaluation of safety in drug development: Design, analysis, and reporting, Q. Jiang and H.A. Xia, Editors. 2015, Chapman & Hall: London. 55-68.

278. Xia HA, Jiang Q. Statistical evaluation of drug safety data. Therapeutic Innovation and Regulatory Science, 2014, 48(1): 109-120.

279. Ioannidis JP. Why most published research findings are false. PLoS Med, 2005, 2(8): e124.

280. Nüesch E, Trelle S, Reichenbach S, Rutjes AW, Tschannen B, Altman DG, Egger M, Juni P. Small study effects in meta-analyses of osteoarthritis trials: meta-epidemiological study. BMJ, 2010, 341: c3515.

281. Moreno SG, Sutton AJ, Thompson JR, Ades AE, Abrams KR, Cooper NJ. A generalized weighting regression-derived meta-analysis estimator robust to small-study effects and heterogeneity. Stat Med, 2012, 31(14): 1407-1417.

282. Kirkham JJ, Altman DG, Williamson PR. Bias due to changes in specified outcomes during the systematic review process. PLoS One, 2010, 5(3): e9810.

283. Trikalinos TA, Churchill R, Ferri M, Leucht S, Tuunainen A, Wahlbeck K, Ioannidis JP, project E-P. Effect sizes in cumulative meta-analyses of mental health randomized trials evolved over time. J Clin Epidemiol, 2004, 57(11): 1124-1130.

284. CIOMS Working Group IX. Practical approaches to risk minimisation for medicinal products: Report of CIOMS Working Group IX. 2014, Geneva, Switzerland: Council for International Organizations of Medical Sciences (CIOMS).

285. European Medicines Agency. Guideline on good pharmacovigilance practices (GVP). Module VI – Management and reporting of adverse reactions to medicinal products (Rev 1) [online]. 2014, 28. http://www.ema.europa.eu/docs/en_GB/document_library/Scientific_guideline/2014/09/WC500172402.pdf.

286. Rezaie A. Absolute Versus Relative Risk: Can We Persuaded by Information Framing? Asian J Epidemiol, 2012, 5: 62-65.

287. European Medicines Agency. Guideline on good pharmacovigilance practices (GVP). Module XV – Safety communication. 2012. http://www.ema.europa.eu/docs/en_GB/document_library/Scientific_guideline/2013/01/WC500137666.pdf.

288. Uppsala Monitoring Centre. Dialogue in pharmacovigilance. 2002.

289. Uppsala Monitoring Centre. Effective communication in pharmacovigilance: the Erice report., in International Conference on Developing Effective Communications in Pharmacovigilance. 1997, Uppsala Monitoring Centre: Erice, Sicily, Italy.

290. Pamer CA, Hammad TA, Wu YT, Kaplan S, Rochester G, Governale L, Mosholder AD. Changes in US antidepressant and antipsychotic prescription patterns during a period of FDA actions. Pharmacoepidemiol Drug Saf, 2010, 19(2): 158-174.

CHAPTER 6.

RESOURCES

Conducting a meta-analysis should be seen as undertaking a major project. Thorough planning, mobilization of expertise and identification of technical resources at the very early stages are critical to achieving a successful outcome. The goal of Chapter 6 is to focus on the resources needed to conduct a meaningful meta-analysis. General references are provided to guide team decision-making, although flexibility is encouraged since the specific question(s) will dictate the expertise needed. In addition to scientific planning, a dedicated team repository is recommended to comply with good clinical practice documentation guidelines. Since the appropriate search strategy and data sources are important criteria for success, this chapter provides introductory guidance along these lines. It is recommended that the scope of a proposed meta-analysis include consideration of public as well as proprietary data sources, as may be appropriate and available.

6.1 The core team – organizational aspects of conducting a meta-analysis

Successfully conducting a meta-analysis requires a diverse range of skills and expertise. Therefore, it is recommended that, in industry, regulatory or academic settings, a core team with appropriate skills should be established to coordinate and ensure that all tasks in the design, conduct and/or evaluation of the meta-analysis are completed and both help and drive actions arising from the final report. While required skills will vary depending on the meta-analysis to be undertaken, it is recommended at a minimum that the meta-analysis team has, or can access, expertise in drug safety, statistics, epidemiology, the relevant clinical field of investigation and general clinical medicine, project management, and information research (e.g. from an experienced specialist librarian). Teams should have the flexibility to draw others into the project as expertise is required (e.g. toxicology, pharmacology, biomarkers, data analysis programming).

One of the first tasks of the core team is to plan the meta-analysis. Details that should be determined as part of the initial planning phase include agreement on the aim or objectives of the meta-analysis, the types of target studies to be included, the databases or other information sources to be searched, target timelines and milestones for the project, the dissemination strategy for the outcome, assignation of tasks and responsibilities, and clarification of communication and reporting lines.

On a practical note, the team should make arrangements for a data repository for all information associated with the meta-analysis and should consider what the record management and transparency requirements of the project are in terms of information to be stored and the use of consistent labelling. With regard to scenarios that involve many trials from several sponsors (as when the request comes from a regulatory body), it is imperative to develop a master data file (a common data model) with clear definitions of the requested variables and the way they are coded [9].

For the analysis, the team should choose the statistical software to be used. This decision should not be based on the results but on the availability of appropriate methods in the software.

6.2 General resources

There are a number of resources to assist a team in planning a meta-analysis. It is important that team members be aware of these and other guidance documents that give advice for appropriate planning and conduct of a meta-analysis.

Cochrane Handbook

The *Cochrane handbook for systematic reviews of interventions* [6] contains detailed information on the process of preparing and maintaining Cochrane systematic reviews on the effects of health-care interventions as well as material on meta-analysis in general.

Agency for Healthcare Research and Quality (AHRQ): *Methods guide for effectiveness and comparative effectiveness reviews*

AHRQ, located within the US Department of Health and Human Services, supports research that helps people make more informed decisions and improves the quality of health-care services. As part of its mission, AHRQ has published a "methods guide" for conducting comparative effectiveness reviews [291].

Institute of Medicine (IOM): *Standards for systematic reviews*

The US Institute of Medicine has published recommended standards for systematic reviews of the comparative effectiveness of medical or surgical interventions with the intention of assuring objective, transparent, and scientifically valid systematic reviews [91].

Enhancing the QUAlity and Transparency Of health Research (EQUATOR [17])

This organization collects resources for writing and publishing health research. It has a comprehensive searchable database of reporting guidelines and also links to other resources relevant to research reporting.

Centre for Reviews and Dissemination (CRD)

CRD in England produced a report that could be useful, entitled *Systematic reviews: CRD's guidance for undertaking reviews in health care* [95].

Preferred Reporting Items for Systematic Reviews and Meta-Analyses (PRISMA)

Several PRISMA statements and checklists have been published. PRISMA checklists mainly contain an evidence-based minimum set of items for reporting on systematic reviews and meta-analyses [18-20, 266, 269]. The PRISMA-P statements also give advice regarding what to include in a protocol [267, 268]

Meta-analysis of observational studies in epidemiology (MOOSE) guidelines

The *MOOSE guidelines* [265] are for meta-analysis and systematic reviews of observational studies.

Annex 1 to the Guide on methodological standards in pharmacoepidemiology (European Medicines Agency)

This document contains guidance on conducting systematic reviews and meta-analyses of completed comparative pharmcoepidemiological studies of safety outcomes, as part of the ENCePP *Guide on methodological standards in pharmacoepidemiology* (http://www.encepp.eu/standards_and_guidances/documents/ENCePP_Methods_Guide_Annex1.pdf).

In the regulatory area it is important for teams to be mindful of any specific requirements of agencies. Both the US FDA and the EMA publish current guidances on their websites. These should be consulted as part of the planning process. For example, as of 2015, EMA guidance was found at EMEA/CHMP: *Points to consider on application with 1. meta-analysis and 2. one pivotal study* [292]. If preparing a meta-analysis for regulatory submission, teams could also consider seeking direct regulatory scientific advice as part of the planning process.

Several publications have discussed various aspects of systematic reviews and meta-analyses of AEs and safety data to some extent [6, 48, 60, 83, 86, 87]. For example, the Cochrane Adverse Effects Methods Group [87] and the Safety Planning, Evaluation and Reporting Team (SPERT), provide specific guidance related to meta-analyses of AEs and safety data [60]. Other pertinent guidance documents include the ICH M4E published by the International Conference on Harmonisation [88], the US Food and Drug Administration's *FDA Guidance on premarketing risk assessment* [89], and the report from CIOMS Working Group VI [59].

6.3   Search strategy and databases

A good search strategy is critical to the success of a meta-analysis. Apart from identification of all potentially relevant and appropriate terms, consideration must be given to the database for searching. There are a number of databases that should be considered. Sponsors and regulatory agencies will have their own internal databases but should additionally be reviewing publicly accessible databases, if available, to capture material collected outside those of the sponsors. The exception to this occurs during the early pre-market period where external data are limited or if a sponsor is requested by a regulator to undertake a meta-analysis of its internal holdings only. Academics and researchers have a choice of databases in the public domain. Some are freely accessible, but for many there is a cost associated with access. Limiting the database search to free sources may not result in the optimal collection of data. There is also increasing willingness and, in some cases, legal obligation to facilitate access to clinical data from regulatory dossiers.

The Medline and Embase databases are leading databases of international literature from the medical sciences. Use of these databases should be regarded as an essential starting point by anyone considering undertaking a meta-analysis.

▶ MEDLINE is a bibliographic database of the US National Library of Medicine (NLM) that contains over 22 million references to journal articles from more than 5500 biomedical journals indexed with NLM Medical Subject Headings (MeSH®). www.nlm.nih.gov/pubs/factsheets/medline.html.

▶ Embase from Elsevier Life Science Solutions is a comprehensive international database of biomedical data with over 28 million records from over 8400 currently published journals. www.elsevier.com/online-tools/embase.

▶ PubMed (MEDLINE) is a web search interface that provides access to over 23 million citations from Medline, life science journals and online books, including links to full-text articles at participating publishers' websites. It is provided free of charge by the US National Center for Biotechnology Information (NCBI). www.ncbi.nlm.nih.gov/pubmed.

▶ The Cochrane Library (including the Cochrane Central Register of Controlled Trials) contains a number of useful resources, including the Cochrane Database of Systematic Reviews (CDSR) and the Cochrane Central Register of Controlled Trials. www.cochranelibrary.com/.

▶ Web of Science (Science Citation Index) is an online subscription-based scientific citation indexing service maintained by Thomson Reuters. Biosis Previews is one of the bibliographic database services on the Thomson Reuters Web of Science research platform. http://wokinfo.com/.

▶ Cumulative Index to Nursing and Allied Health Literature (CINAHL) provides indexing of the top nursing and allied health literature covering a wide range of topics, including nursing, biomedicine, health sciences librarianship, alternative/complementary medicine, consumer health and 17 allied health disciplines. https://health.ebsco.com/products/the-cinahl-database.

▶ PsycINFO® is an abstracting and indexing database devoted to peer-reviewed literature in the behavioural sciences and mental health. www.apa.org/pubs/databases/psycinfo/index.aspx.

▶ POPLINE is a free resource, maintained by the Knowledge for Health (K4Health) Project at the Johns Hopkins Bloomberg School of Public Health/Center for Communication Programs and is funded by the United States Agency for International Development (USAID). POPLINE includes information on population and family planning, specifically research in contraceptive methods, family planning services, research in human fertility, maternal and child health, HIV/AIDS in developing countries, programme operations and evaluation, demography, and other related health, law and policy issues. www.k4health.org/k4health-products#POPLINE.

▶ LILACS is a comprehensive index of scientific and technical literature of Latin America and the Caribbean. http://lilacs.bvsalud.org/en/.

▶ African Index Medicus (AIM), produced by the World Health Organization, in collaboration with the Association for Health Information and Libraries in Africa (AHILA), is an international index to African health literature and information sources. http://indexmedicus.afro.who.int/.

▶ WHO Global Health Library (GHL) is a WHO initiative as part of its strategy of knowledge management in global public health. www.who.int/library/en/.

▶ ProQuest's Sociological Abstracts database abstracts and indexes the international literature in sociology and related disciplines in the social and behavioural sciences. www.proquest.com/libraries/academic/databases/sociology.html.

▶ ClinicalTrials.gov is a service of the US National Institutes of Health. It is a registry and results database of publicly and privately supported clinical studies of human participants conducted around the world. The site was originally created as a repository for clinical trial protocols, but now also contains clinical trial results summaries.

▶ The European Union Clinical Trials Registry is hosted by the European Medicines Agency (EMA) and contains information on clinical trials in the European Union (EU) member states and the European Economic Area (EEA), as well as clinical trials which are conducted outside the EU/EEA if they form part of a paediatric investigation plan (PIP). www.clinicaltrialsregister.eu/

▶ ISRCTN is a registry and curated database containing the basic set of data items deemed essential to describe a study at inception, according to the requirements set out by the WHO International Clinical Trials Registry Platform (ICTRP) and the International Committee of Medical Journal Editors (ICMJE) guidelines. All study records in the database are freely accessible and searchable and have been assigned an ISRCTN ID. The registry was launched in 2000 in response to the growing body of opinion in favour of prospective registration of RCTs. Originally ISRCTN stood for 'International Standard Randomized Controlled Trial Number'; however, over the years the scope of the registry has widened beyond randomized controlled trials to include any study designed to assess the efficacy of health interventions in a human population. This includes both observational and interventional trials. Current Controlled Trials was a website operated by Current Controlled Trials Limited which allowed users to search, register and share information about RCTs. This is now affiliated with BioMedCentral. www.controlled-trials.com/

▶ International Clinical Trials Registry Platform (ICTRP) is a WHO database for voluntary registration of clinical trials and publication of an internationally-agreed set of information about the design, conduct and administration of clinical trials. http://apps.who.int/trialsearch/

The development and access to databases suitable for meta-analysis is dynamic. The above listed suggestions are not definite and will change over time. They provide a repertoire of possible options, with all their intrinsic opportunities, challenges and limitations. None of the suggestions are necessarily more important than the others. The team should discuss different feasible scenarios for databases to be used for a meta-analysis but should also consider predefined alternatives.

References Chapter 6

6. Higgins JPT, Green S, eds. Cochrane Handbook for Systematic Reviews of Interventions Version 5.1.0 [updated March 2011]. 2011, The Cochrane Collaboration. http://handbook.cochrane.org/.

9. Hammad TA, Laughren T, Racoosin J. Suicidality in pediatric patients treated with antidepressant drugs. Arch Gen Psychiatry, 2006, 63(3): 332-339.

17. EQUATOR Enhancing the QUAlity and Transparency Of health Research. A comprehensive searchable database of reporting guidelines. www.equator-network.org.

18. Moher D, Liberati A, Tetzlaff J, Altman DG, PRISMA Group. Preferred reporting items for systematic reviews and meta-analyses: the PRISMA statement. J Clin Epidemiol, 2009, 62(10): 1006-1012.

19. Stewart LA, Clarke M, Rovers M, Riley RD, Simmonds M, Stewart G, Tierney JF, Group P-ID. Preferred Reporting Items for Systematic Review and Meta-Analyses of individual participant data: the PRISMA-IPD Statement. JAMA, 2015, 313(16): 1657-1665.

20. Hutton B, Salanti G, Caldwell DM, Chaimani A, Schmid CH, Cameron C, Ioannidis JP, Straus S, Thorlund K, Jansen JP, Mulrow C, Catala-Lopez F, Gotzsche PC, Dickersin K, Boutron I, Altman DG, Moher D. The PRISMA extension statement for reporting of systematic reviews incorporating network meta-analyses of health care interventions: checklist and explanations. Ann Intern Med, 2015, 162(11): 777-784.

48. Hammad TA, Pinheiro SP, Neyarapally GA. Secondary use of randomized controlled trials to evaluate drug safety: a review of methodological considerations. Clin Trials, 2011, 8(5): 559-570.

59. CIOMS Working Group VI. Management of Safety Information from Clinical Trials. 2005, Geneva: Council for International Organizations of Medical Sciences.

60. Crowe BJ, Xia HA, Berlin JA, Watson DJ, Shi H, Lin SL, Kuebler J, Schriver RC, Santanello NC, Rochester G, Porter JB, Oster M, Mehrotra DV, Li Z, King EC, Harpur ES, Hall DB. Recommendations for safety planning, data collection, evaluation and reporting during drug, biologic and vaccine development: a report of the safety planning, evaluation, and reporting team. Clin Trials, 2009, 6(5): 430-440.

83. Golder S, McIntosh HM, Loke Y. Identifying systematic reviews of the adverse effects of health care interventions. BMC Med Res Methodol, 2006, 6: 22.

86. Huang HY, Andrews E, Jones J, Skovron ML, Tilson H. Pitfalls in meta-analyses on adverse events reported from clinical trials. Pharmacoepidemiol Drug Saf, 2011, 20(10): 1014-1020.

87. Loke YK, Price D, Herxheimer A, Group CAEM. Systematic reviews of adverse effects: framework for a structured approach. BMC Med Res Methodol, 2007, 7: 32.

88. ICH International Conference on Harmonisation. ICH M4E Guideline on Enhancing the Format and Structure of Benefit-Risk Information in ICH. 2014. http://www.ich.org/products/ctd/ctdsingle/article/revision-of-m4e-guideline-on-enhancing-the-format-and-structure-of-benefit-risk-information-in-ich.html.

89. U.S. Food and Drug Administration. Guidance for Industry: Premarketing Risk Assessment. 2012. http://www.fda.gov/downloads/RegulatoryInformation/Guidances/UCM126958.pdf.

91. Institute of Medicine. Finding What Works in Health Care: Standards for Systematic Reviews. 2011, Washington, DC: The National Academies Press.

95. Centre for Reviews and Dissemination. Systematic reviews: CRD's guidance for undertaking reviews in health care. 2009. www.york.ac.uk/media/crd/Systematic_Reviews.pdf.

265. Stroup DF, Berlin JA, Morton SC, Olkin I, Williamson GD, Rennie D, Moher D, Becker BJ, Sipe TA, Thacker SB. Meta-analysis of observational studies in epidemiology: a proposal for reporting. Meta-analysis Of Observational Studies in Epidemiology (MOOSE) group. JAMA, 2000, 283(15): 2008-2012.

266. Liberati A, Altman DG, Tetzlaff J, Mulrow C, Gøtzsche PC, Ioannidis JP, Clarke M, Devereaux PJ, Kleijnen J, Moher D. The PRISMA statement for reporting systematic reviews and meta-analyses of studies that evaluate health care interventions: explanation and elaboration. PLoS Med, 2009, 6(7): e1000100.

267. Moher D, Shamseer L, Clarke M, Ghersi D, Liberati A, Petticrew M, Shekelle P, Stewart LA, PRISMA-P Group. Preferred reporting items for systematic review and meta-analysis protocols (PRISMA-P) 2015 statement. Syst Rev, 2015, 4: 1.

268. Shamseer L, Moher D, Clarke M, Ghersi D, Liberati A, Petticrew M, Shekelle P, Stewart LA, Group P-P. Preferred reporting items for systematic review and meta-analysis protocols (PRISMA-P) 2015: elaboration and explanation. BMJ, 2015, 349: g7647.

269. Zorzela L, Loke YK, Ioannidis JP, Golder S, Santaguida P, Altman DG, Moher D, Vohra S. PRISMA harms checklist: improving harms reporting in systematic reviews. BMJ, 2016, DOI: http://dx.doi.org/10.1136/bmj.i157. http://www.bmj.com/content/352/bmj.i157.

291. AHRQ Agency for Healthcare Research and Quality. Methods Guide for Effectiveness and Comparative Effectiveness Reviews. 2014. http://effectivehealthcare.ahrq.gov/ehc/products/60/318/CER-Methods-Guide-140109.pdf.

292. European Medicines Agency. Points to consider on application with 1. meta-analyses; 2. one pivotal study. 2001. http://www.ema.europa.eu/docs/en_GB/document_library/Scientific_guideline/2009/09/WC500003657.pdf.

APPENDIX 1.

CASE STUDY – ANTIDEPRESSANTS AND SUICIDAL EVENTS IN ADULTS

Summary of main points and questions demonstrated by this example

This example:

▶ demonstrates issues related to evaluating a drug class problem;

▶ explains the prospective analysis plan of retrospective data including pre-specified hypothesis, inclusion criteria, outcomes measures, master data file and analysis;

▶ provides examples of uniform, retrospective, and blinded adjudication of outcomes;

▶ explains how to deal with methods issues such as stratification by trial for effect estimation with sparse outcome data;

▶ shows use of patient-level data to explore subgroups and hazard pattern over time;

▶ raises considerations to statistical significance, multiple testing of consistent findings, and type I and type II errors;

▶ underscores issues around the need for regulatory action based on sometimes limited information (e.g. on some drugs within a class of drugs).

1. Background

Patients with depression are at substantially increased risk of suicide [293]. Antidepressants are marketed on the basis of their ability to reduce measures of depression. Conversely, speculation about a possible association of antidepressants with suicide has existed for several decades based on anecdotal evidence. In 1991 the US FDA held an advisory committee meeting to review the risk of suicidal events and selective serotonin reuptake inhibitors, a class of commonly-used antidepressants. The committee concluded that there was insufficient evidence for causality. In 2003, a manufacturer of an antidepressant provided the FDA with data suggesting an association of the drug with suicidal-related events among paediatric patients. The FDA expanded its review of the association to all antidepressants studied in paediatric populations and conducted a meta-analysis which consisted of 24 trials with 4582 patients. There was a statistically significant effect of the antidepressants relative to placebo for the composite outcome of suicidal behaviour and ideation [9]. It should be stressed that there were no completed suicides in these trials. On the basis of this finding and advice from an external advisory committee, the FDA added a boxed warning to the package inserts for all classes of antidepressants. Subsequently, the FDA conducted a meta-analysis of adult patients [271]. Additional details for this example can be found in a publicly available briefing package from the US FDA [294].

2. Meta-analyses story

The US FDA meta-analysis employed a pre-specified written analysis plan, which specified trial inclusion criteria, hypotheses, outcome definitions, master data file (a common data model) with clear definitions of the requested variables as well as the way they are coded, analysis methods, sensitivity analyses and subgroups.

The FDA requested data on all completed double-blind, randomized, placebo-controlled trials of at least 20 patients conducted by manufacturers of antidepressants. An additional requirement was that patient-level data were available. Basing the meta-analysis on trials available to drug makers, in addition to other available trials, has some important advantages. For example, the trial set does not suffer from publication bias, because publication has no bearing on the inclusion of the trials. Also, because of regulatory requirements, trials from drug manufacturers often contain detailed patient-level data that include medical history, baseline characteristics, patient dispositions, patient outcomes and AEs. In addition, focusing on the relatively small group of drug manufacturers (nine) allowed for the timely acquisition of the large amounts of pertinent data. Overall, the meta-analysis obtained data on 372 trials with usable data. Most trials were relatively short-term in duration (12 weeks or less).

It was important to create uniform high-quality outcome measures. The outcomes of interest, suicidal behaviour and ideation events, were typically not captured actively and consistently in the trials, as these events were not the primary focus of the trials. The FDA provided instructions to the drug manufacturers on a plan for a retrospective identification and adjudication of events. Using AE data, potential events were identified with a specified algorithm including text searches of coded and verbatim AE terms and comment fields. From these events, narratives of the events were created. On the basis of narratives of the events that were blinded to exposure status, qualified personnel classified the events into specific outcomes including completed suicide, attempted suicide, preparatory actions toward imminent suicidal behaviours, or suicidal ideation utilizing the Columbia Classification Algorithm for Suicide Assessment (C-CASA) [82]. The algorithm has been shown to have high reliability so the overall process resulted in outcome measures that were consistently defined across trials and patients.

The primary endpoint was suicide behaviour and ideation, representing the first four categories of the C-CASA classification, and the primary analysis population was all studies conducted in major depressive disorder, other depression disorders, and other psychiatric disorders. Secondary analysis considered other groups of indications. Only events occurring during treatment or within one day of stopping treatment were included in the analysis.

The primary analysis was a fixed-effect "exact" method for a stratified OR, stratified by study [295]. This provided estimates of the OR vs. placebo. The methods used for the estimation of the drug effect in the meta-analysis were chosen to both maintain the within-trial comparisons and to perform well with low events rates. Without maintaining the within-trial comparisons, the overall estimate may not reflect the true effect because of differences in background rates and allocation ratios among the trials. To maintain the within-trial comparison, the estimation method was stratified by trial. Some statistical estimators and their uncertainty measures require large sample sizes. This was a concern in the antidepressant meta-analysis in which the rate of outcome events was low.

Several sensitivity and supporting analyses were performed to explore the robustness of the primary analysis. Differences in exposure and observational time between the randomized-treatment arms within trials were explored to ensure that differences could not explain any observed drug effect. Heterogeneity of the drug effect across trials was explored graphically and statistically. The results of a random-effects method were compared to the primary method, which was a fixed-effect method. The results between the two methods were found to be similar, suggesting that different weighting of the trials did not change the overall findings. The primary analysis method implicitly did not make use of trials without events. To examine the consequences of including these trials, a stratified RD estimator was used. This method makes use of trials without any events. Again, qualitatively the two methods produced similar findings.

Subgroups were examined for consistency and, because of direct clinical interests, were based on age, gender, geographical location and setting of care.

The meta-analysis found that the overall association of antidepressant drugs and suicidal behaviour and ideation was not statistically significant, which is in contrast to the findings of the FDA meta-analysis of paediatric patients. However, the association was nearly statistically significant for young adults and the meta-analysis showed a clear pattern in the association as related to patient age (see Figure A.1). The inclusion of the result from the paediatric meta-analysis supported this trend. Note that statistical significance was not adjusted for multiple testing of subgroups, in spite of the fact that there were clearly many subgroups explored. In drug safety in general, because of the potential harm involved, the possible error of falsely detecting an adverse effect when there is no effect had to be balanced with the possible error of falsely not detecting an adverse effect when there is an effect.

3. Action

The FDA sought advice from a meeting of the FDA Advisory Committees on the interpretation and possible regulatory actions based on the findings of the meta-analysis. The FDA chose to update the boxed warning to warn about the risk of suicidal behaviour and ideation associated with antidepressants for young adult patients in addition to paediatric patients. The need for close observation during the initiation of treatment was emphasized. This was done despite the fact that the overall effect was not statistically significant, and no age subgroup showed a statistically harmful effect. The decision was based on the consistency of the age trend as seen in Figure A.1 and on the consistency with the paediatric results. The warning states that the effect was not seen in patients over the age of 24, and for patients aged 65 and older the risk may be reduced. It should be noted that it was the clear pattern in the effect as related to patient age and not statistical significance that led to the warning.

The FDA chose to update the label on all classes of antidepressant drugs, including those not studied in the meta-analysis. The rationale for this decision was that the effect was seen in most drugs in the analysis and, because the mechanism of the effect was not known, the FDA could not determine which drugs would or would not be affected. The warning also noted that the effect was based on information from short-term trials. No conclusion was made for the effect beyond short-term use.

Motivated by the experiences with the meta-analyses of the antidepressants and other drug classes, the FDA produced a draft guidance document on the prospective collection of suicidal events in clinical trials [81]. The guidance promotes specific prospective collection of suicidal events with the aims of: (1) better recognizing and treating patients with events during the trials, and (2) better detecting and estimating an adverse effect of the drug on suicidal events.

At the European Medicines Agency, a review was performed by its Pharmacovigilance Working Party (now the Pharmacovigilance Risk Assessment Committee, known as "PRAC") for the Committee for Medicinal Products for Human Use (CHMP), reaching similar conclusions to those of the FDA. National agencies were recommended to add a boxed warning, to notify patients and caregivers of the risk and to monitor closely, especially during initiation of therapy. In children it is specifically emphasized not to use these drugs outside the approved indications.

In Japan, following the reported results of the meta-analysis of adult patients by the FDA, labelling of all antidepressants was updated and the risk of suicidal ideation and suicide attempt in the patients aged 24 years or younger was described in the precautions for indication.

Figure A.1 FDA meta-analysis showing odds ratios by age group for suicidal behavior and ideation (psychiatric indications)

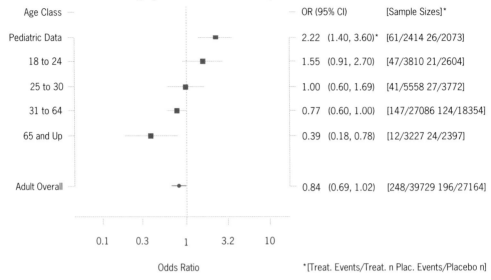

Age Class	OR (95% CI)	[Sample Sizes]*
Pediatric Data	2.22 (1.40, 3.60)*	[61/2414 26/2073]
18 to 24	1.55 (0.91, 2.70)	[47/3810 21/2604]
25 to 30	1.00 (0.60, 1.69)	[41/5558 27/3772]
31 to 64	0.77 (0.60, 1.00)	[147/27086 124/18354]
65 and Up	0.39 (0.18, 0.78)	[12/3227 24/2397]
Adult Overall	0.84 (0.69, 1.02)	[248/39729 196/27164]

Odds Ratio   *[Treat. Events/Treat. n Plac. Events/Placebo n]

Source: US FDA. Referenced in FDA Memo November 16, 2006: Briefing document for Psycho-pharmacologic Drugs Advisory Committee, December 13, 2006. www.fda.gov/ohrms/dockets/ac/06/briefing/2006-4272b1-01-FDA.pdf, within which is referenced US FDA Statistical Evaluation of Suicidality in Adults Treated with Antidepressants, Date of Review: November 17, 2006, Levenson & Holland, Div of Biometrics and Psychiatric Products, Figure 6, page 38, a re-analysis of Hammad's "Relationship between psychotropic drugs and pediatric suicidality." US FDA, 16 August 2004. [81] Used with permission.

References Appendix 1

9.   Hammad TA, Laughren T, Racoosin J. Suicidality in pediatric patients treated with antidepressant drugs. Arch Gen Psychiatry, 2006, 63(3): 332-339.

81.   U.S. Food and Drug Administration. Guidance for Industry: Suicidal Ideation and Behavior: Prospective Assessment of Occurrence in Clinical Trials, August 2012, accessed at. 2012. http://www.fda.gov/drugs/guidancecomplianceregulatoryinformation/guidances/ucm315156.htm.

82.   Posner K, Oquendo MA, Gould M, Stanley B, Davies M. Columbia Classification Algorithm of Suicide Assessment (C-CASA): classification of suicidal events in the FDA's pediatric suicidal risk analysis of antidepressants. Am J Psychiatry, 2007, 164(7): 1035-1043.

271.   Stone M, Laughren T, Jones ML, Levenson M, Holland PC, Hughes A, Hammad TA, Temple R, Rochester G. Risk of suicidality in clinical trials of antidepressants in adults: analysis of proprietary data submitted to US Food and Drug Administration. BMJ, 2009, 339: b2880.

293.   Sadock BJ, Sadock VA, Ruiz P, Kaplan HI. Kaplan & Sadock's comprehensive textbook of psychiatry. 9th ed. 2009, Philadelphia: Wolters Kluwer Health/Lippincott Williams & Wilkins.

294.   U.S. Food and Drug Administration. FDA briefing document for the December 13, 2007 Psychopharmacologic Drugs Advisory Committee meeting. 2007. http://www.fda.gov/ohrms/dockets/ac/06/briefing/2006-4272b1-index.htm.

295.   Gart JL. Point and interval estimation of the common odds ratio in the combination of 2 × 2 tables with fixed marginals. Biometrika, 1970, 57: 471-475.

APPENDIX 2.

CASE STUDY – ERYTHROPOIETIN STIMULATING AGENTS AND THROMBOEMBOLIC EVENTS IN ONCOLOGY SETTING

Summary of main points and questions demonstrated by this example

This example:

▶ notes that heterogeneity of populations/design is common, but a small value for the global test of heterogeneity (or I^2) does not rule out the possibility that there is a (potential) specific source of heterogeneity of treatment effects;

▶ shows that it can be difficult to distinguish between random variability and the idea that the "meta-analysis masks a signal in individual studies";

▶ underscores the need to be careful interpreting results when the endpoint being examined is not a primary (or secondary) endpoint but was only collected as an AE (and asks whether this is as much of a consideration when the endpoint is mortality as when the endpoint is something less serious);

▶ considers how to treat studies that have different lengths of follow-up;

▶ discusses what studies should be included in a meta-analysis;

▶ discusses which population should be studied for a certain AE of interest.

1. Background

Erythropoiesis-stimulating agents (ESAs) increase haemoglobin concentrations, reduce the need for red blood cell transfusions, and could reduce symptoms of anaemia, such as fatigue, in patients with cancer. However, in recent years, several publications (see Table A.2) have reported that these drugs may increase the risk of thromboembolic events and it has been speculated that they might stimulate tumour growth. Uncertainty remains about whether and how these drugs affect survival. Potential adverse effects have also been identified in patients with chronic kidney disease. However, to keep the focus on a single population in the interest of avoiding unnecessary complexity, we limit consideration here to studies of cancer patients with anaemia. The study by Leyland-Jones [296], known as the BEST study, initiated ESA treatment at higher haemoglobin levels and treated patients to higher target haemoglobin levels than is currently recommended in label guidance for ESAs, and continued treatment for as long as a year. This study was the first to give rise to concerns about potentially increased mortality.

.

2. Meta-analyses story

A number of systematic reviews and meta-analyses have been published to address the question of whether mortality is increased by ESA administration in the oncology setting. Several of these studies are summarized in Table A.2. Rather than describe each of the meta-analyses in any detail, we note here some specific aspects relating to these meta-analyses and the lessons learned.

During the whole story there was a constant debate about the inclusion criteria of studies in the meta-analyses in terms of duration of follow-up. Some comments at the US FDA Advisory Committee meetings recommended including only those studies with "adequate survival follow-up". In this context, it is important to note the early separation of the survival curves (by four months of follow-up) in the BEST study and in other studies within the first few months of follow-up. This suggests that any effect on survival could occur early in follow-up, so the notion of "adequate" – presumably longer – follow-up is of questionable importance. Further, it is important to note that BEST is among the first, largest and most important studies raising concern. Thus, in a sense, the signal of concern that one wishes to confirm or rule out is an early survival signal. It is also of note that the survival curves in the BEST study converge after about 12 months of follow-up, so that an analysis of longer-term follow-up yields a mortality hazard ratio close to unity. Thus, the short-term analysis was actually more sensitive with regard to safety, and the long-term follow-up would have actually risked missing the early survival difference altogether. In any case, practitioners of meta-analysis and methodologists who study the technique generally advocate inclusion of all information provided by randomized comparisons, regardless of the duration of follow-up, as long as ascertainment of deaths is complete. Further, studies with a small number of deaths will not contribute much information to a meta-analysis, and will be "down-weighted" in any summary statistics.

In most of the studies, mortality was not a primary endpoint. This raises the question of completeness of ascertainment of deaths, when they are collected only as AEs and not as study endpoints. This raises yet a further question of whether a "hard" endpoint, such as death, needs to be a study endpoint in order to be considered valid. Mortality events can be ascertained, with some effort, from sources outside the trials. This might increase the validity of studies of mortality as an endpoint, although the additional follow-up could delay obtaining an answer to urgent safety questions.

Heterogeneity of findings seemed to be a key issue in virtually all the meta-analyses conducted. The values of I-squared (I^2) in the meta-analyses were either 0% or close to 0%. Nonetheless, some patterns of variability seemed somewhat consistent across meta-analyses. Thus:

a) Studies in patients with anaemia of cancer show a consistently elevated relative risk, as do studies of radiation therapy. Analyses limited to studies of chemotherapy-induced anaemia show consistently lower relative risks, although the extent to which that is true varies from meta-analysis to meta-analysis.

b) When examined at the study level (but not in the Bohlius analysis when stratifying on patient-level baseline haemoglobin) [297], studies with lower mean baseline haemoglobin tend to show lower relative risks.

c) Target haemoglobin is less compelling as a stratification factor than baseline haemoglobin. It is important to distinguish between the target haemoglobin (i.e. the level of haemoglobin that is defined as the intended therapeutic goal of the ESA treatment) and the achieved haemoglobin level (i.e. the actual value attained during treatment). In targeting a high haemoglobin value, dose might be increased in patients who do not respond early on with an increase in achieved haemoglobin.

d) In the 2006 AHRQ analysis [297], and in an early version of the Bennett paper (when it was presented as a poster) [298], stratification by "within-label" vs. "off-label" suggested that the studies "within-label" show a lower relative risk. Sensitivity analyses that have been conducted by excluding the BEST study (because it was clearly off-label use of ESA, as noted above) show relative risks close to 1.0 (generally around 1.03–1.05, with CIs overlapping 1.0).

3. Action

The safety of these drugs has been the subject of numerous hearings and regulatory label interventions of the US FDA at Advisory Committee meetings and of the European Medicines Agency, essentially directed at restriction of use and risk minimization.

Table A.2 Published systematic reviews and meta-analyses that address the question of whether mortality is increased by ESA administration in the oncology setting

First author (year)	Journal	Number of studies	Number of subjects	Findings
Glaspy (2010)# [299]	Br J Cancer	60	15 323 total hemotherapy: 12 108	Mortality (60 studies): OR=1.06 (95% CI: 0.97–1.15; I^2 = 0%) Mortality, chemotherapy only (47 studies): OR = 1.03 (95% CI: 0.93–1.13; I^2 = 1.2%) Mortality, chemotherapy, BEST removed: OR = 0.98 (0.89, 1.09) VTE (44 studies): OR=1.48 (95% CI: 1.28–1.72)
Bohlius (2009)* [297]	Lancet	53	13 933 total chemotherapy: 10 441	Hazard ratio [HR]: 1.17 (95% CI: 1.06–1.30; I^2 = 0%) Chemotherapy (38 trials): 1.10 (0.98–1.24) Chemotherapy, BEST removed: 1.03 (0.90,1.18)
Bennett (2008) [298]	JAMA	51	13 611	HR: 1.10 (95% CI: 1.01-1.20) Chemotherapy: 1.09 (0.99–1.19), I^2 = 21%
Tonelli (2009) [300]	CMAJ	52 28 (mortality analysis, 31 comparisons)	12 006 total 6525 (for analysis of total mortality)	[RR] 1.15 (95% CI: 1.03 to 1.29; I^2 = 0%)

Sponsor authors included.

* Based on individual patient-level data.

Abbreviations: VTE = venous thromboembolism; HR = hazard ratio; OR = odds ratio; CI = confidence interval; RR = risk ratio.

Source: Created by CIOMS X 2016.

References Appendix 2

296. Leyland-Jones B, BEST Investigators and Study Group. Breast cancer trial with erythropoietin terminated unexpectedly. Lancet Oncol, 2003, 4(8): 459-460.

297. Bohlius J, Wilson J, Seidenfeld J, Piper M, Schwarzer G, Sandercock J, Trelle S, Weingart O, Bayliss S, Brunskill S, Djulbegovic B, Benett CL, Langensiepen S, Hyde C, Engert E. Erythropoietin or darbepoetin for patients with cancer. Cochrane Database Syst Rev, 2006(3): CD003407.

298. Bennett CL, Silver SM, Djulbegovic B, Samaras AT, Blau CA, Gleason KJ, Barnato SE, Elverman KM, Courtney DM, McKoy JM, Edwards BJ, Tigue CC, Raisch DW, Yarnold PR, Dorr DA, Kuzel TM, Tallman MS, Trifilio SM, West DP, Lai SY, Henke M. Venous thromboembolism and mortality associated with recombinant erythropoietin and darbepoetin administration for the treatment of cancer-associated anemia. JAMA, 2008, 299(8): 914-924.

299. Glaspy J, Crawford J, Vansteenkiste J, Henry D, Rao S, Bowers P, Berlin JA, Tomita D, Bridges K, Ludwig H. Erythropoiesis-stimulating agents in oncology: a study-level meta-analysis of survival and other safety outcomes. Br J Cancer, 2010, 102(2): 301-315.

300. Tonelli M, Hemmelgarn B, Reiman T, Manns B, Reaume MN, Lloyd A, Wiebe N, Klarenbach S. Benefits and harms of erythropoiesis-stimulating agents for anemia related to cancer: a meta-analysis. CMAJ, 2009, 180(11): E62-71.

APPENDIX 3.

CASE STUDY – TIOTROPIUM AND CARDIOVASCULAR EVENTS IN COPD PATIENTS

Summary of main points and questions demonstrated by this example

This example:

▶ shows methodological challenges with some published meta-analyses of trials about drug safety;

▶ considers how to deal with discrepancies in meta-analyses of several small trials and one large trial;

▶ underscores the need for the use of measured restraint during evaluations of some meta-analyses in order to ensure that the use of the investigated drug is not restricted in a way that unnecessarily denies beneficial interventions to patients who need them; and

▶ demonstrates that publication in high-impact journals might not be an automatic surrogate for the strength of the evidence (given that several streams of evidence might exist for a particular safety signal, findings from published post-hoc meta-analyses should be taken within this context and initially treated as "preliminary" evidence until these findings are verified with other streams of evidence).

1. Background

Chronic obstructive pulmonary disease (COPD) is a leading cause of death worldwide with no current drug therapy that can alter the progressive decline in lung function associated with the disease. In 2004, the US FDA approved the use of tiotropium delivered by the HandiHaler device, the first long-acting anticholinergic bronchodilator for treatment of COPD. Trials supporting the approval of tiotropium demonstrated sustained bronchodilation over a 24-hour period (i.e. symptomatic relief, but still not a disease-altering therapy) [128]. However, concerns have been raised about tiotropium's safety by a meta-analysis published in 2008 [15].

2. Meta-analyses story

In September 2008, Singh et al. published in *JAMA* a meta-analysis of 17 randomized clinical trials evaluating the cardiovascular risk associated with inhaled anticholinergic agents. The study reported a relative risk of cardiovascular events of 1.60 (95% CI: 1.22–2.10) for inhaled anticholinergics (including trials of tiotripium and ipratropium, each compared with controls). The study concluded that the use of inhaled anticholinergics was associated with a significantly increased risk of major adverse cardiovascular events, including death from cardiovascular causes, myocardial infarction and stroke [15, 301].

Shortly afterwards, the Understanding Potential Long-Term Impacts on Function with Tiotropium (UPLIFT) trial was published in the *New England Journal of Medicine* and did not show the previously reported increased risk (death from cardiovascular causes: RR 0.73 (95% CI: 0.56–0.95) [128]. UPLIFT was a large, four-year RCT where data on deaths, including the vital status of patients who withdrew from the study, were collected prospectively, and the cause of death was adjudicated by an independent committee. With 17 721 patient-years of exposure, the size of the UPLIFT study surpassed the size of all the trials that were used in the previously published meta-analysis [302].

Review by the FDA underscored methodological limitations in the Singh et al. meta-analysis that may explain the disparities between its findings and the UPLIFT study:

These [methodological limitations] included: potentially biased study selection, which was limited to trials reporting cardiovascular events; lack of assessment of patient follow-up time, with no accounting for differential discontinuation rates, which were significantly higher among patients given placebo (patients who continue to take placebo may be generally healthier than those who stop taking it, and potential differences in baseline cardiovascular risk factors were not accounted for in the analysis); lack of information on occurrence of AEs in patients who withdrew from many of the included trials; lack of patient-level data; and the fact that trials on short-acting and long-acting anticholinergics were combined in the main analysis. In contrast, the UPLIFT trial had a large sample size, a long follow-up period and pre-specified safety endpoints, including all AEs, serious AEs and death from any cause. Information on vital status was collected for 97% of treated patients until the end of treatment day 1440, and for 75% of treated patients until off treatment follow-up day 1470. Findings regarding stroke, cardiovascular events and death were consistent across a variety of analyses [128].

3. Action

The FDA convened a meeting of the Pulmonary–Allergy Drugs Advisory Committee (known as "PADAC") on 19 November 2009, to discuss the data on cardiovascular risk and mortality associated with the exposure to the drug. The PADAC decided that the data from UPLIFT adequately addressed the potential stroke or cardiovascular signals. Because of the strength of the UPLIFT data and the potential methodological limitations of the Singh meta-analysis, the FDA concluded that current evidence does not support the conclusion that there is an increased risk of stroke, heart attack or death associated with tiotropium [303].

References Appendix 3

15. Singh S, Loke YK, Furberg CD. Inhaled anticholinergics and risk of major adverse cardiovascular events in patients with chronic obstructive pulmonary disease: a systematic review and meta-analysis. JAMA, 2008, 300(12): 1439-1450.

128. Michele TM, Pinheiro S, Iyasu S. The safety of tiotropium–the FDA's conclusions. N Engl J Med, 2010, 363(12): 1097-1099.

301. Erratum J. Incorrect data in: Inhaled anticholinergics and risk of major adverse cardiovascular events in patients with chronic obstructive pulmonary disease: a systematic review and meta-analysis. JAMA, 2009, 301(12): 1227-1230.

302. Tashkin DP, Celli B, Senn S, Burkhart D, Kesten S, Menjoge S, Decramer M, Investigators US. A 4-year trial of tiotropium in chronic obstructive pulmonary disease. N Engl J Med, 2008, 359(15): 1543-1554.

303. U.S. Food and Drug Administration. Early communication about an ongoing safety review of tiotropium [marketed as Spiriva HandiHaler]. 2008. http://www.fda.gov/Drugs/DrugSafety/PostmarketDrugSafetyInformationforPatientsandProviders/DrugSafetyInformationforHeathcareProfessionals/ucm070651.htm.

APPENDIX 4.

CASE STUDY – ROSIGLITAZONE AND CARDIOVASCULAR EVENTS IN DIABETES PATIENTS

Summary of main points demonstrated by this example

This example demonstrates:

▶ challenges in conducting a meta-analysis when outcomes of interest are not primary or secondary outcomes of the trials;

▶ having a pre-specified systematic review protocol with pre-specified analysis plan helps avoid post-hoc analysis;

▶ many small trials in a meta-analysis, taken collectively, can have a large weight, or even a higher weight, than larger trials designed for those outcomes (the small trials will inevitably not have been designed to study outcomes that occur infrequently, which is a motivation for doing systematic review and meta-analysis);

▶ sensitivity analyses are important, given that different methods can provide different answers.

1. Background

Patients with type II diabetes – also known as non-insulin-dependent diabetes mellitus (or "NIDDM") or adult-onset diabetes – are known to be at high risk of cardiovascular disease (CVD), and especially myocardial infarction (MI). Their obvious disorders of glucose metabolism have led many to assume that reduction in blood glucose levels (glycaemic control) would result in a reduction in CVD, and especially MIs. However, when the newer agents such as rosiglitazone were introduced, there was little evidence that such an effect existed, even for older, established drugs. There was reasonably good evidence that lowering blood glucose levels would reduce microvascular complications (e.g. retinopathy, potentially leading to blindness), but little evidence regarding their impact on macrovascular complications such as MI.

Drugs like rosiglitazone (a class of drugs known as thiazolidinediones) were first approved in the USA in 1999 and in Europe (as second-line drugs) in 2000. They were licensed for NIDDM on the basis of their glycaemic control benefits.

It was notable that this class of drugs showed increases in fluid retention and in body weight, which would work against any CVD benefit, notably congestive heart failure and MIs. It should also be noted that, initially at least, in the EU rosiglitazone was contraindicated for use in combination with insulin, and in patients with congestive heart failure.

2. Meta-analyses story

In 2007, Nissen & Wolski published a meta-analysis in the New England Journal of Medicine [13]. The meta-analysis considered 116 trials, of which 42 met their inclusion criteria. There were two large trials included ("DREAM" and "ADOPT"), but most trials were rather small. The results were, for myocardial infarction, an OR of 1.43 (95% CI: 1.03–1.98; $P = 0.03$), and for death from cardiovascular causes, an OR of 1.64 (95% CI: 0.98–2.74; $P = 0.06$). Although criteria on inclusions and exclusions were set out in the paper, no mention is made of a protocol focusing on particular CVD outcomes.

The analysis method used was Peto's (fixed-effect) method, which may be argued as suitable for rare events. This and similar methods cannot use trials with zero events in both arms, so four trials did not contribute to the analysis of MIs and 19 did not contribute to the deaths from CVD. Twenty-one of the 38 trials used for MI had only a single event and 15 of the 23 trials used for the analysis of CVD death also had a single event. Of the 21 trials with a single event, 16 had the event reported on rosiglitazone and five on the comparator treatment.

Several other features of the meta-analysis are of note. First, the authors reported that, for those trials where rosiglitazone was combined with insulin and compared with insulin alone, the OR was 2.78 (95% CI: 0.58–13.3, $P = 0.20$). If these trials are excluded, the overall results for MI and for death lose their statistical significance. This is not simply a product of reduced statistical power (because there are fewer events in the sub-analysis) but also of an OR estimate that was closer to the null. Of note, the initial approval of rosiglitazone in the EU included a contraindication for use with insulin, although this contraindication was later removed. The ORs for other comparators ranged from 1.14 (95% CI: 0.70–1.86, $P = 0.59$) for metformin to 1.80 (95% CI: 0.95–3.39), $P = 0.07$ for placebo.

Second, in some analyses, the trials with a small number of events, when taken collectively, have as much or more weight in the meta-analysis as either of the two large trials. This is understandable since the small trials had 44 MIs and 25 deaths from CVD reported for rosiglitazone; the two large trials collectively reported 42 MIs and 14 deaths from CVD for rosiglitazone, indicating a substantial contribution of the small trials to the analysis. Looking specifically at the weights contributed to the analyses, for ORs, ADOPT contributed 41% of the weight to the Peto analysis, DREAM contributed 17%, and the small trials contributed 42% of the weight.

A further trial, RECORD (Rosiglitazone evaluated for cardiovascular outcomes) [304], designed and powered to examine composite CVD outcomes, including MI as part of the composite, had an interim analysis carried out in response to the Nissen & Wolski publication, and was published soon after their NEJM paper. The interim analysis found, for the primary composite endpoint of hospitalization or death from cardiovascular causes, a hazard ratio [HR] of 1.08; 95% CI: 0.89–1.31. For MI, in an analysis that included both adjudicated and non-adjudicated events, they found an HR of 1.23 (0.81–1.86), $P = 0.34$. At one of the FDA Advisory Committee meetings on this topic (http://www.fda.gov/downloads/AdvisoryCommittees/CommitteesMeetingMaterials/Drugs/EndocrinologicandMetabolicDrugsAdvisoryCommittee/UCM222628.pdf) one scientist from the FDA was highly critical of the design and conduct of this study, despite the study having been designed specifically to collect adjudicated CVD events.

Subsequent to the Nissen & Wolski (2007) manuscript, additional meta-analyses as well as additional analyses based on the same dataset were published with varying conclusions (some agreed with the original findings while some concluded that there was inadequate evidence that either MI or CVD death rates were increased). For a list of some of these, see references in Böhning et al. [305]). Nissen & Wolski published an update in 2010 [306] drawing similar conclusions to those in their 2007 paper.

3. Action

In 2007, regulators worldwide issued warnings about cardiovascular risk and reiterated warnings around the congestive heart failure associated with fluid retention. This was also emphasized in the report on the RECORD trial.

In 2010, the FDA further restricted its use to existing patients or to second-line use. In Europe, at the European Medicines Agency, a further review took place in 2010 and rosiglitazone was suspended across the EU, and it has not been marketed there since then and remains unavailable in 2016.

At the end of 2013, the FDA removed most of the restrictions on rosiglitazone saying it does "not show an increased risk of heart attack compared to the standard type 2 diabetes medicines metformin and sulfonylurea" based on additional review of the final results of the dedicated cardiovascular outcome trial. As of 16 December 2015 the FDA had removed the final remaining restrictions placed on the use of rosiglitazone (http://www.medscape.com/viewarticle/856056).

References Appendix 4

[13.] Nissen SE, Wolski K. Effect of rosiglitazone on the risk of myocardial infarction and death from cardiovascular causes. N Engl J Med, 2007, 356(24): 2457-2471.
[304.] Home PD, Pocock SJ, Beck-Nielsen H, Gomis R, Hanefeld M, Jones NP, Komajda M, McMurray JJ, RECORD Study Group. Rosiglitazone evaluated for cardiovascular outcomes–an interim analysis. N Engl J Med, 2007, 357(1): 28-38.
[305.] Böhning D, Mylona K, Kimber A. Meta-analysis of clinical trials with rare events. Biom J, 2015, 57(4): 633-648.
[306.] Nissen SE, Wolski K. Rosiglitazone revisited: an updated meta-analysis of risk for myocardial infarction and cardiovascular mortality. Arch Intern Med, 2010, 170(14): 1191-1201.

ANNEX I. GLOSSARY

1. Bias

A systematic deviation in results from the truth.

Source: Proposed by CIOMS X.

2. Censored/censoring

An observation is said to be censored in time when the event of interest cannot be observed at the time at which the analysis is conducted. Special cases are right censoring when the observation has not yet been observed at the time of the analysis, left censoring when the observation occurred sometime before the observation period began, and interval censoring when the observation's time of occurrence has been recorded as within a time interval.

Source: Proposed by CIOMS X.

3. Channelling

A situation where drugs are prescribed to patients differentially based on the presence or absence of factors prognostic of patient outcomes.

Source: Guidance for Industry and FDA Staff: "Best Practices for Conducting and Reporting Pharmacoepidemiologic Safety Studies Using Electronic Healthcare Data," U.S. Food and Drug Administration, Center for Biologics and Evaluation and Research, Drug Safety, May 2013.

4. Composite endpoint

A composite endpoint is a single measure of effect, based on a combination of individual endpoints, each component being itself clinically meaningful. An example of a composite endpoint is MACE (Major Adverse Cardiac Event) which is typically a combination of cardiovascular death, non-fatal myocardial infarction and non-fatal stroke.

Source: Proposed by CIOMS X.

5. Confounding

Confounding occurs when a variable exists that influences the use of a drug or medical procedure (or its avoidance) and also alters the probability of an outcome, the association of which to the drug or procedure is under investigation.

Source: Adapted from Boston University School of Public Health, MPH modules, ©2016, definition of confounding, http://sphweb.bumc.bu.edu/otlt/MPH-Modules/BS/BS704-EP713_Confounding-EM/.

6. Confounding by indication

Confounding by indication is a type of confounding bias that occurs when a symptom or sign of disease is judged as an indication (or a contraindication) for a given therapy, and is therefore associated both with use of drug or medical procedure (or its avoidance) and with a higher probability of an outcome related to the disease for which the drug is indication (or contraindicated).

Source: Miquel Porta, ed (2014) A Dictionary of Epidemiology (sixth ed.) Oxford University Press. ISBN-13: 978-0199976737.

7. Covariate

A variable that is possibly predictive of the outcome under study. A covariate may be of direct interest to the study or it may be a confounding variable or effect modifier.

Source: Miquel Porta, ed (2014) A Dictionary of Epidemiology (sixth ed.) Oxford University Press. ISBN-13: 978-0199976737.

8. Crude pooling

A method of combining data from a number of studies that ignores which study they came from, treating them as if they came from a single study.

Source: Proposed by CIOMS X.

9. Cumulative meta-analysis

A meta-analysis in which studies are added one at a time in a specified order (e.g. according to date of publication or quality) and the results are summarized as each new study is added. In a graph of a cumulative meta-analysis, each horizontal line represents the summary of the results as each study is added, rather than the results of a single study.

Source: Glossary of Terms in The Cochrane Collaboration. Available from http://community.cochrane. org/organizational-info/resources.

10. Ecological bias (also known as ecological fallacy)

An erroneous inference that may occur because an association observed between variables on an aggregate level does not necessarily represent or reflect the association that exist at an individual level.

Source: Miquel Porta, ed (2014) A Dictionary of Epidemiology (sixth ed.) Oxford University Press. ISBN-13: 978-0199976737.

11. Effect modifier

A feature of study individuals such that a treatment or risk factor has different effect at different levels of the feature, i.e. that there is an interaction between the feature and the treatment. The term is mostly used in an epidemiological context.

Source: Dodge, Y, The Oxford Dictionary of Statistical Terms,6th ed., International Statistical Institute, New York. Oxford University Press, Inc., 2006.

12. Endpoint

An endpoint ("target" variable, outcome) is a measurement specified and designed to be capable of capturing the clinically relevant effects of an intervention, and to provide convincing evidence directly related to a specific objective of the meta-analysis.

Source: Proposed by CIOMS X. Adapted from ICH International Conference on Harmonisation. ICH E9 Statistical principles for clinical trials ICH Harmonised Tripartite Guideline. 1995.

13. Fixed effects

Fixed effects refer to one way in which the individual study estimates of treatment effect are combined in the meta-analysis. In a fixed-effect model the variability among the individual study estimates is not included in the analysis. The contribution of each study is usually determined only by the precision of each study. (See also Random effects #22.)

Source: Proposed by CIOMS X.

14. Forest plot

A forest plot is a graphical representation of the individual results of each study included in a meta-analysis together with the combined meta-analysis result. The plot also allows readers to see the heterogeneity among the results of the studies. The results of individual studies are shown as squares centred on each study's point estimate. The weight of the study in the overall analysis is often represented by the area of a square plotted at the point estimate. A horizontal line runs through each square to show each study's CI - usually, but not always, a 95% CI. The overall estimate from the meta-analysis and its CI are shown at the bottom, often represented as a diamond. The centre of the diamond represents the pooled point estimate, and its horizontal tips represent the CI.

Proposed CIOMS X in modification of Cochrane definition. (Source: Glossary of Terms in the Cochrane Collaboration. Available from http://community.cochrane.org/organizational-info/resources.)

15. Heterogeneity

Heterogeneity refers to differences among studies and/or study results. Heterogeneity can generally be classified in three ways: clinical heterogeneity, methodological heterogeneity and statistical heterogeneity [252]. Clinical heterogeneity refers to differences among trials in their patient selection (e.g. disease conditions under investigation, eligibility criteria, patient characteristics, or geographical differences), interventions (e.g. duration, dosing, nature of the control) and outcomes (e.g. definitions of endpoints, follow-up duration, cut-off points for scales). Methodological heterogeneity refers to the differences in study design (e.g. the mechanism of randomization) and in study conduct (e.g. allocation concealment, blinding, extent and handling of withdrawals and loss to follow up, or analysis methods). Decisions about what constitutes clinical heterogeneity and methodological heterogeneity do not involve any calculation and are based on judgement. On the other hand, statistical heterogeneity represents a notion that individual studies may have results that are not numerically consistent with each other, and the variation is more than what is expected on the basis of sampling variability alone. Statistical heterogeneity may be caused by known clinical and methodological differences among trials, by unknown trial (clinical or methodological) characteristics, or it may be due to chance.

Source: Proposed by CIOMS X. Adapted from: 1) Thompson SG. Why sources of heterogeneity in meta-analysis should be investigated. BMJ, 1994, 309(6965)and 2) Berlin JA, Crowe BJ, Whalen E, Xia HA, Koro CE, Kuebler J. Meta-analysis of clinical trial safety data in a drug development program: answers to frequently asked questions. Clin Trials, 2013.

16. Individual participant data

Data that list the values of variables in the study grouped so that a set of values from a single participant can be identified. This term contrasts with summary level data in which all results are presented as functions of the individual participant data from which values pertaining to an individual cannot be retrieved by any further calculation.

Source: Proposed by CIOMS X. Adapted from The European Network of Centres for Pharmacoepidemiology and Pharmacovigilance (ENCePP). Annex 1 to the Guide on Methodological Standards in Pharmacoepidemiology, 17 December 2015, EMA/686352/201. Available at http://www.encepp.eu/standards_and_guidance.

17. Meta-analysis

The statistical combination of quantitative evidence from two or more studies to address common research questions, where the analytical methods appropriately take into account that the data are derived from multiple individual studies.

Source: Proposed by CIOMS X.

18. Meta-regression

A technique used in meta-analysis to explore the relationship between study characteristics (e.g. concealment of allocation, baseline risk, timing of the intervention) and study results (the magnitude of effect observed in each study) in a systematic review.

Source: Glossary of Terms in the Cochrane Collaboration. Available from http://community.cochrane.org/organizational-info/resources.

19. Odds ratio

The ratio of one "odds" divided by another, where the "odds" of an event is a proportion divided by one minus the proportion. The way that it is commonly estimated from sample data is illustrated in Annex II. Glossary case study.

Source: Proposed by CIOMS X

20. Outcome

Synonym for Endpoint (see #12). See also "Composite endpoint" (#4).

Source: Proposed by CIOMS X.

21. Primary endpoint

The primary endpoint is the endpoint or outcome that defines the primary objective of a meta-analysis. (See also: Endpoint, Composite endpoint, Outcome.)

Source: Proposed by CIOMS X.

22. Random effects

Random effects refers to one of the two ways in which the individual study estimates of treatment effect are combined in the meta-analysis. In a random-effects meta-analysis model the variability among the individual study estimates is included in the analysis. Thus, the contribution of each study to the overall estimate is usually determined by both the precision within each study and the among-study variability. (See also Fixed effects.)

Source: Proposed by CIOMS X.

23. Relative risk

A general term used to refer to relative measures of the magnitude of effect of the intervention or risk factor on the outcome, such as hazard ratio, odds ratio, risk ratio or rate ratio.

Source: Proposed by CIOMS X.

24. Risk difference

The difference between two proportions. The way that it is commonly estimated from sample data is illustrated in Annex II. Glossary case study.

Source: Proposed by CIOMS X.

25. Risk ratio

The ratio of one proportion to another. The way that it is commonly estimated from sample data is illustrated in Annex II. Glossary case study.

Source: Proposed by CIOMS X.

26. Sensitivity analysis

An analysis used to determine how sensitive the results of a study or systematic review are to changes in how it was done. Sensitivity analyses are used to assess how robust the results are to uncertain decisions or assumptions about the data and the methods that were used.

Source: Glossary of Terms in the Cochrane Collaboration. Available from http://community.cochrane.org/organizational-info/resources.

27. Sequential meta-analysis

A particular form of a cumulative meta-analysis accounting for multiple testing in which clinical trials can be stopped early (or planned future trials could be stopped before they start) based on interim analyses or sequential analyses. In principle, sequential analyses can also be used to decide whether enough evidence has been gathered in completed trials to make further trials unnecessary.

Source: Proposed by CIOMS X.

28. Summary-level data

Refers to summary statistics (e.g. mean, standard deviation) at the level of a group of participants (e.g. treatment and control group) in a single study.

Source: Proposed by CIOMS X.

29. Systematic review

A review of a clearly formulated question that uses systematic and explicit methods to identify, select and critically appraise relevant research, and to collect and analyse data from the studies that are included in the review. Statistical methods (meta-analysis) may or may not be used to analyse and summarize the results of the included studies.

Source: Glossary of Terms in The Cochrane Collaboration. Available from http://community.cochrane. org/organizational-info/resources.

30. Trial

An experiment in which two or more interventions, one of which could be a control intervention or "usual care", are compared by being randomly allocated to participants. In most trials, one intervention is assigned to each individual but sometimes assignment is to specific groups of individuals (e.g. in a household) or interventions are assigned within individuals (e.g. in different orders or to different parts of the body).

Source: Proposed by CIOMS X.

31. Weight

The weight of an individual study estimate of treatment effect is the relative amount that the study-specific estimate contributes to the estimation of the overall treatment effect. The weights in a fixed-effect model are often determined by the inverse of the within-study variance and in a random-effects model by the inverse of the within-study plus among-study variance. However, there is no necessary connection between the weights of the individual study estimates and fixed-effect or random-effects models. The choice of weights can be informed by other considerations.

Source: Proposed by CIOMS X.

GLOSSARY CASE STUDY – MEASURES OF EFFECT IN HORMONE REPLACEMENT THERAPY AND BREAST CANCER

This annex to the glossary presents a straightforward case study of how common meta-analysis statistical measures are calculated, to illustrate the definitions of the risk ratio (RR), risk difference (RD) and odds ratio (OR). A randomized clinical trial comparing combined hormone replacement therapy (HRT) with placebo, known as the Women's Health Initiative (WHI) trial, was carried out in the USA. A key outcome was invasive breast cancer with the results shown in the table below which comes from Table 2 of Rossouw et al. [307].

Results

Over 16 000 women were randomized and followed up for an average of 5.2 years. The numbers with and without breast cancer are given in the table below.

Treatment group	With breast cancer	Without breast cancer	Total
HRT	166	8340	8506
Placebo	124	7978	8102

Risk is the number who have an event (in this case breast cancer) divided by the number who could have had that event. Here the risk of breast cancer in the HRT intervention group (166/8506) = 0.0195 which is often presented as 1.95%. It is a proportion or a percentage. The risk of breast cancer in the placebo group is (124/8102) = 0.0153 [1.53%].

The RR usually has the treated group as a numerator and the comparison group as the denominator = 0.0195/0.0153 = 1.275. The RD = 0.0195 - 0.0153 = 0.0042, or 0.42% or 4.2 per 1000.

An alternative to proportions are the odds. The odds of breast cancer in those on HRT are 166/8340 = 0.0199. The denominator is now those who did not have the event. The odds of breast cancer for those on placebo is 124/7978 = 0.0155.

The odds are higher than the risks, but with fairly rare events the odds are fairly similar to the risks. The OR is the ratio of these odds = .0199/.0155 = 1.280. Again this is similar to the RR (because the event is rare), with the note that the OR is further from unity (1) than the RR. An RR and an OR of 1 both suggest no difference between the groups.

References glossary case study

252. Thompson SG. Why sources of heterogeneity in meta-analysis should be investigated. BMJ, 1994, 309(6965): 1351-1355.

307. Rossouw JE, Anderson GL, Prentice RL, LaCroix AZ, Kooperberg C, Stefanick ML, Jackson RD, Beresford SA, Howard BV, Johnson KC, Kotchen JM, Ockene J, Writing Group for the Women's Health Initiative I. Risks and benefits of estrogen plus progestin in healthy postmenopausal women: principal results From the Women's Health Initiative randomized controlled trial. JAMA, 2002, 288(3): 321-333.

MEMBERSHIP AND MEETINGS OF THE CIOMS X WORKING GROUP

The CIOMS Working Group X on Evidence Synthesis and Meta-Analysis for Drug Safety met in a series of eight meetings from June 2011 through September 2014 with a final Editorial Meeting in July 2015. This Working Group report was reviewed in draft form by participating members in June and following a review by the editorial team and team members was finalized thereafter for publication. The members of the Editorial Team were: Brenda Crowe (Editor-in-Chief), Jesse Berlin, Tarek Hammad, Bert Leufkens, and Tongtong Wang, supported by Gunilla Sjölin-Forsberg and Karin Holm. The chapter leads were Stephen Evans (Ch. 2), William Gregory (Ch. 1), Leonie Hunt (Ch. 6), George Rochester (first stage Ch. 3 and 4), Tongtong Wong (second stage Ch. 3 and 4), and David Wright (Ch. 5).

During the course of its work, the Working Group recognized its membership to represent the following broad groups of stakeholders (or interested parties) in risk minimization approaches: regulatory authorities; biopharmaceutical industry; international organizations; and academia. Members, their institutional affiliations and stakeholder groups (as defined above) as well as a chronological summary of the Working Group meetings are listed below.

Name	Organization (Stakeholder group)	Duration of membership*
Ando, Yuki	MHLW/PMDA, Japan (Regulatory authority)	Partial
Arguinzoniz, Miguel	Roche (Pharma industry)	Full
Asano, Kunihito	MHLW/PMDA, Japan (Regulatory authority)	Partial
Berlin, Conny	Novartis (Pharma Industry)	Full
Berlin, Jesse	Johnson & Johnson (Pharma industry)	Full
Boddy, Alexander	Sanofi Aventis S.A. (Pharma industry)	Full
Brueckner, Andreas	Novartis (Pharma Industry)	Full
Cochino, Emil	European Medicines Agency (Regulatory authority)	Partial
Cogo, Elise	Health Canada (Regulatory authority)	Partial
Crowe, Brenda	Eli Lilly and Company (Pharma industry)	Full
Evans, Stephen	London School of Hygiene and Tropical Medicine (Academia)	Full

Name	Organization (Stakeholder group)	Duration of membership*
Gaffney, Michael	Pfizer *(Pharma industry)*	Full
Gregory, William	Pfizer *(Pharma industry)*	Full
Hammad, Tarek	Merck *(Pharma industry 2014-2015)*; US FDA Regulatory authority 2012-2013	Full
Hobbiger, Stephen	GSK *(Pharma industry)*	Full
Heaton, Stephen	Bayer HealthCare *(Pharma industry)*	Full
Hunt, Leonie	TGA, Australia *(Regulatory authority)*	Full
Idänpään-Heikkilä, Juhana	CIOMS (Senior Adviser, Past Secretary-General) *(International organization)*	Full
Irs, Alar	World Health Organization *(International organization)*	Partial
Koh, Yvonne	HSA Singapore *(Regulatory authority)*	Partial
Leufkens, Bert	CBG-MEB, Netherlands *(Regulatory authority)*	Full
Levenson, Mark	US Food and Drug Administration *(Regulatory authority)*	Partial
Liteplo, Robert	Health Canada *(Regulatory authority)*	Partial
Michel, Alexander	Bayer HealthCare *(Pharma industry)*	Full
Quartey, George	Roche *(Pharma industry)*	Full
Rägo, Lembit	World Health Organization *(International organization)*	Partial
Rochester, George	US Food and Drug Administration *(Regulatory authority)*	Partial
Shah, Arvind	Merck *(Pharma industry)*	Full
Sjölin-Forsberg, Gunilla	CIOMS (Secretary-General, 2010-2015) *(International organization)*	Full
Slattery, Jim	European Medicines Agency *(Regulatory authority)*	Full
Strassmann, Valerie	BfArM, Germany *(Regulatory authority)*	Full
Straus, Sabine	CBG-MEB, Netherlands *(Regulatory authority)*	Partial
Uyama, Yoshiaki	MHLW/PMDA, Japan *(Regulatory authority)*	Partial
Wang, Tongtong	Health Canada 2012-2014 *(Regulatory authority)*	Full
Wright, David	MHRA, United Kingdom *(Regulatory authority)*	Full
Xia, H. Amy	Amgen *(Pharma industry)*	Full
Yoshida, Michihiro	Takeda *(Pharma industry)*	Full

* "Partial" denotes membership in the Working Group for a portion of the three-year period while «Full» denotes membership and active participation for the full period.

CIOMS X Working Group meetings**

Date	Location	Host
June 2011	Geneva, Switzerland	CIOMS
November 2011	Geneva, Switzerland	CIOMS
March 2012	Silver Spring, Maryland, USA	FDA
September 2012	London, UK	EMA
March 2013	Utrecht, Netherlands	MEB
September 2013	Singapore	HSA
February 2014	Durham, North Carolina, USA	GSK
September 2014	Basel, Switzerland	Novartis
July 2015 (Editorial Team)	New Brunswick, New Jersey, USA	J&J

** Costs for travel and accommodation were covered by each Working Group member's parent organization *or by CIOMS as per rules*, and were not covered by the meeting hosts.

BIBLIOGRAPHICAL REFERENCES

1.   Google. Keyword "meta-analysis" searched 26 March 2015. www.google.com.

2.   U.S. National Center for Biotechnology Information. PubMed advanced search builder; keyword "meta-analysis" searched 26 March 2015. http://www.ncbi.nlm.nih.gov/pubmed/advanced.

3.   European Medicines Agency. ICH guideline E2C (R2) on periodic benefit-risk evaluation report (PBRER). 2013, EMA/CHMP/ICH/544553/1998, 1-45. http://www.ema.europa.eu/docs/en_GB/document_library/Regulatory_and_procedural_guideline/2012/12/WC500136402.pdf.

4.   Borenstein M, Hedges LV, Higgins JP, Rothstein HR. Introduction to Meta-analysis. 2009, Chichester, UK: John Wiley & Sons.

5.   Egger M, Smith GD, Altman D. Systematic reviews in health care: meta-analysis in context. 2nd ed. 2008, London, UK: John Wiley & Sons.

6.   Higgins JP, Green S, eds. Cochrane Handbook for Systematic Reviews of Interventions Version 5.1.0 [updated March 2011]. 2011, The Cochrane Collaboration. http://handbook.cochrane.org/.

7.   Khan K, Kunz R, Kleijnen J, Antes G. Systematic reviews to support evidence-based medicine. , 2011. 2nd ed. 2011, London, UK: Royal Society of Medicine.

8.   U.S. Food and Drug Administration. Guidance for industry: Diabetes mellitus-evaluating cardiovascular risk in new antidiabetic therapies to treat Type 2 diabetes. 2008. http://www.fda.gov/downloads/Drugs/GuidanceComplianceRegulatoryInformation/Guidances/UCM071627.pdf.

9.   Hammad TA, Laughren T, Racoosin J. Suicidality in pediatric patients treated with antidepressant drugs. Arch Gen Psychiatry, 2006, 63(3): 332-339.

10.   Kim PW, Wu YT, Cooper C, Rochester G, Valappil T, Wang Y, Kornegay C, Nambiar S. Meta-analysis of a possible signal of increased mortality associated with cefepime use. Clin Infect Dis, 2010, 51(4): 381-389.

11.   McMahon AW, Levenson MS, McEvoy BW, Mosholder AD, Murphy D. Age and risks of FDA-approved long-acting beta(2)-adrenergic receptor agonists. Pediatrics, 2011, 128(5): e1147-1154.

12.   Colman E, Szarfman A, Wyeth J, Mosholder A, Jillapalli D, Levine J, Avigan M. An evaluation of a data mining signal for amyotrophic lateral sclerosis and statins detected in FDA's spontaneous adverse event reporting system. Pharmacoepidemiol Drug Saf, 2008, 17(11): 1068-1076.

13.   Nissen SE, Wolski K. Effect of rosiglitazone on the risk of myocardial infarction and death from cardiovascular causes. N Engl J Med, 2007, 356(24): 2457-2471.

14.   Nissen SE. Setting the RECORD straight. JAMA, 2010, 303(12): 1194-1195.

15.   Singh S, Loke YK, Furberg CD. Inhaled anticholinergics and risk of major adverse cardiovascular events in patients with chronic obstructive pulmonary disease: a systematic review and meta-analysis. JAMA, 2008, 300(12): 1439-1450.

16.   Varas-Lorenzo C, Riera-Guardia N, Calingaert B, Castellsague J, Salvo F, Nicotra F, Sturkenboom M, Perez-Gutthann S. Myocardial infarction and individual nonsteroidal anti-inflammatory drugs meta-analysis of observational studies. Pharmacoepidemiol Drug Saf, 2013, 22(6): 559-570.

17.   EQUATOR Enhancing the QUAlity and Transparency Of health Research. A comprehensive searchable database of reporting guidelines. www.equator-network.org.

18.   Moher D, Liberati A, Tetzlaff J, Altman DG, PRISMA Group. Preferred reporting items for systematic reviews and meta-analyses: the PRISMA statement. J Clin Epidemiol, 2009, 62(10): 1006-1012.

19.   Stewart LA, Clarke M, Rovers M, Riley RD, Simmonds M, Stewart G, Tierney JF, Group P-ID. Preferred Reporting Items for Systematic Review and Meta-Analyses of individual participant data: the PRISMA-IPD Statement. JAMA, 2015, 313(16): 1657-1665.

20.   Hutton B, Salanti G, Caldwell DM, Chaimani A, Schmid CH, Cameron C, Ioannidis JP, Straus S, Thorlund K, Jansen JP, Mulrow C, Catala-Lopez F, Gotzsche PC, Dickersin K, Boutron I, Altman DG, Moher D. The PRISMA extension statement for reporting of systematic reviews incorporating network meta-analyses of health care interventions: checklist and explanations. Ann Intern Med, 2015, 162(11): 777-784.

21.   Chalmers I, Hedges LV, Cooper H. A brief history of research synthesis. Eval Health Prof, 2002, 25(1): 12-37.

22.   Glass GV. Primary, Secondary, and Meta-Analysis of Research. Educ Res, 1976, 5, 3-8. http://www.jstor.org/stable/1174772.

23. Baber NS, Lewis JA. Beta-blockers in the treatment of myocardial infarction. BMJ, 1980, 281(6232): 59.

24. Cochrane Collaboration. Cochrane Adverse Effects Methods Group. 2007, The Group aims to develop the methods for producing high quality systematic reviews and to advise the Cochrane Collaboration on how the validity and precision of systematic reviews can be improved. http://aemg.cochrane.org/.

25. Berlin JA, Golub RM. Meta-analysis as evidence: building a better pyramid. JAMA, 2014, 312(6): 603-606.

26. Eysenck HJ. Meta-analysis and its problems. BMJ, 1994, 309(6957): 789-792.

27. Shapiro S. Meta-analysis/Shmeta-analysis. Am J Epidemiol, 1994, 140(9): 771-778.

28. Ioannidis JP, Evans SJ, Gotzsche PC, O'Neill RT, Altman DG, Schulz K, Moher D, Group C. Better reporting of harms in randomized trials: an extension of the CONSORT statement. Ann Intern Med, 2004, 141(10): 781-788.

29. Hodkinson A, Kirkham JJ, Tudur-Smith C, Gamble C. Reporting of harms data in RCTs: a systematic review of empirical assessments against the CONSORT harms extension. BMJ open, 2013, 3(9): e003436.

30. Kearney PM, Baigent C, Godwin J, Halls H, Emberson JR, Patrono C. Do selective cyclo-oxygenase-2 inhibitors and traditional non-steroidal anti-inflammatory drugs increase the risk of atherothrombosis? Meta-analysis of randomised trials. BMJ, 2006, 332(7553): 1302-1308.

31. McGettigan P, Henry D. Cardiovascular risk and inhibition of cyclooxygenase: a systematic review of the observational studies of selective and nonselective inhibitors of cyclooxygenase 2. JAMA, 2006, 296(13): 1633-1644.

32. Hammad TA, Graham DJ, Staffa JA, Kornegay CJ, Dal Pan GJ. Onset of acute myocardial infarction after use of non-steroidal anti-inflammatory drugs. Pharmacoepidemiol Drug Saf, 2008, 17(4): 315-321.

33. Oxford University. Cancer Epidemiology Unit. 2015. http://www.ceu.ox.ac.uk/team/valerie-beral.

34. Collaborative Group on Hormonal Factors in Breast Cancer. Breast cancer and hormonal contraceptives: collaborative reanalysis of individual data on 53 297 women with breast cancer and 100 239 women without breast cancer from 54 epidemiological studies. Lancet, 1996, 347(9017): 1713-1727.

35. Beral V, Banks E, Reeves G, Wallis M. Hormone replacement therapy and high incidence of breast cancer between mammographic screens. Lancet, 1997, 349(9058): 1103-1104.

36. Collaborative Group on Hormonal Factors in Breast C. Familial breast cancer: collaborative reanalysis of individual data from 52 epidemiological studies including 58,209 women with breast cancer and 101,986 women without the disease. Lancet, 2001, 358(9291): 1389-1399.

37. International Collaboration of Epidemiological Studies of Cervical C, Appleby P, Beral V, Berrington de Gonzalez A, Colin D, Franceschi S, Goodhill A, Green J, Peto J, Plummer M, Sweetland S. Cervical cancer and hormonal contraceptives: collaborative reanalysis of individual data for 16,573 women with cervical cancer and 35,509 women without cervical cancer from 24 epidemiological studies. Lancet, 2007, 370(9599): 1609-1621.

38. Lièvre M, Cucherat M, Leizorovicz A. Pooling, meta-analysis, and the evaluation of drug safety. Curr Control Trials Cardiovasc Med, 2002, 3(1): 6.

39. Chuang-Stein C, Beltangady M. Reporting cumulative proportion of subjects with an adverse event based on data from multiple studies. Pharmaceut Statist, 2011, 10(1): 3-7.

40. European Medicines Agency. ICH guideline E2F on development safety update report. 2010. http://www.ema.europa.eu/docs/en_GB/document_library/Scientific_guideline/2010/09/WC500097061.pdf.

41. ICH International Conference on Harmonisation. ICH E9 Statistical principles for clinical trials ICH Harmonised Tripartite Guideline. 1995. http://www.ich.org/products/guidelines/efficacy/efficacy-single/article/statistical-principles-for-clinical-trials.html.

42. ISIS-4 (International Study of Infarct Survival). ISIS-4: a randomised factorial trial assessing early oral captopril, oral mononitrate, and intravenous magnesium sulphate in 58,050 patients with suspected acute myocardial infarction. ISIS-4 (Fourth International Study of Infarct Survival) Collaborative Group. Lancet, 1995, 345(8951): 669-685.

43. ISIS-3 (International Study of Infarct Survival). ISIS-3: a randomised comparison of streptokinase vs tissue plasminogen activator vs anistreplase and of aspirin plus heparin vs aspirin alone among 41,299 cases of suspected acute myocardial infarction. ISIS-3 (Third International Study of Infarct Survival) Collaborative Group. Lancet, 1992, 339(8796): 753-770.

44. ISIS-2 (International Study of Infarct Survival). Randomised trial of intravenous streptokinase, oral aspirin, both, or neither among 17,187 cases of suspected acute myocardial infarction: ISIS-2. ISIS-2 Second International Study of Infarct Survival) Collaborative Group. Lancet, 1988, 2(8607): 349-360.

45.   ISIS-1 (International Study of Infarct Survival). Randomised trial of intravenous atenolol among 16 027 cases of suspected acute myocardial infarction: ISIS-1. First International Study of Infarct Survival Collaborative Group. Lancet, 1986, 2(8498): 57-66.

46.   Fourth International Study of Infarct Survival: protocol for a large simple study of the effects of oral mononitrate, of oral captopril, and of intravenous magnesium. ISIS-4 collaborative group. Am J Cardiol, 1991, 68(14): 87D-100D.

47.   Hammad TA, Neyarapally GA, Iyasu S, Staffa JA, Dal Pan G. The future of population-based postmarket drug risk assessment: a regulator's perspective. Clin Pharmacol Ther, 2013, 94(3): 349-358.

48.   Hammad TA, Pinheiro SP, Neyarapally GA. Secondary use of randomized controlled trials to evaluate drug safety: a review of methodological considerations. Clin Trials, 2011, 8(5): 559-570.

49.   Kalil AC. Is cefepime safe for clinical use? A Bayesian viewpoint. J Antimicrob Chemother, 2011, 66(6): 1207-1209.

50.   Institute of Medicine. Discussion Framework for Clinical Trial Data Sharing: Guiding Principles, Elements, and Activities. 2014, Washington, DC: The National Academies Press.

51.   Olson S, Downey AS, Institute of Medicine (U.S.). Forum on Drug Discovery Development and Translation, Institute of Medicine (U.S.). Forum on Neuroscience and Nervous System Disorders, National Cancer Policy Forum (U.S.), Institute of Medicine (U.S.). Roundtable on Translating Genomic-Based Research for Health, Institute of Medicine (U.S.). Board on Health Sciences Policy, Institute of Medicine (U.S.). Board on Health Care Services. Sharing clinical research data : workshop summary. 2013, Washington, D.C.: The National Academies Press.

52.   Institute of Medicine. Sharing Clinical Trial Data: Maximizing Benefits, Minimizing Risk. 2015. http://iom.nationalacademies.org/Reports/2015/Sharing-Clinical-Trial-Data.aspx.

53.   Wellcome Trust. ClinicalStudyDataRequest.com. 2014, The Wellcome Trust has taken responsibility for managing the review of research proposals and the operation of the Independent review panel (IRP). The Trust will also administer the IRP secretariat and appoint new panel members. www.wellcome.ac.uk. https://www.clinicalstudydatarequest.com/.

54.   Yale School of Medicine. Yale University Open Data Access (YODA) Project. 2015. http://yoda.yale.edu/welcome-yoda-project.

55.   Pharmaceutical Research and Manufacturers of America (PhRMA). PhRMA Principles For Responsible Clinical Trial Data Sharing. 2013. http://www.phrma.org/phrmapedia/responsible-clinical-trial-data-sharing.

56.   European Federation of Pharmaceutical Industries and Associations (EFPIA). Joint Principles for Responsible Clinical Trial Data Sharing to Benefit Patients. 2013. http://transparency.efpia.eu/clinical-trials.

57.   European Medicines Agency. European Medicines Agency policy on publication of clinical data for medicinal products for human use. 2014. http://www.ema.europa.eu/docs/en_GB/document_library/Other/2014/10/WC500174796.pdf.

58.   European Medicines Agency. Questions and answers on the European Medicines Agency policy on publication of clinical data for medicinal products for human use. 2015. http://www.ema.europa.eu/docs/en_GB/document_library/Report/2014/10/WC500174378.pdf.

59.   CIOMS Working Group VI. Management of Safety Information from Clinical Trials. 2005, Geneva: Council for International Organizations of Medical Sciences.

60.   Crowe BJ, Xia HA, Berlin JA, Watson DJ, Shi H, Lin SL, Kuebler J, Schriver RC, Santanello NC, Rochester G, Porter JB, Oster M, Mehrotra DV, Li Z, King EC, Harpur ES, Hall DB. Recommendations for safety planning, data collection, evaluation and reporting during drug, biologic and vaccine development: a report of the safety planning, evaluation, and reporting team. Clin Trials, 2009, 6(5): 430-440.

61.   Hammad TA, Neyarapally GA. Legislative Policy [BJC1] and Science Considerations in the Era of Patient-Centeredness, Big Data, and Value. in Benefit-Risk Assessment Methods in Medicinal Product Development: Bridging Qualitative and Quantitative Assessments, 1st. 2016, CRC Press Taylor and Francis Group: Boca Raton, FL.

62.   Higgins JPT, Altman DG, Gotzsche PC, Juni P, Moher D, Oxman AD, Savovic J, Schulz KF, Weeks L, Sterne JA, Cochrane Bias Methods G, Cochrane Statistical Methods G. The Cochrane Collaboration's tool for assessing risk of bias in randomised trials. BMJ, 2011, 343: d5928.

63.   Bero L. Editorial: Why the Cochrane risk of bias tool should include funding source as a standard item. 2013. http://www.cochranelibrary.com/editorial/10.1002/14651858.ED000075.

64. Sterne JA. Editorial: Why the Cochrane risk of bias tool should **not** include funding source as a standard item. 2013. http://www.cochranelibrary.com/editorial/10.1002/14651858.ED000076.

65. Al-Marzouki S, Roberts I, Evans S, Marshall T. Selective reporting in clinical trials: analysis of trial protocols accepted by The Lancet. Lancet, 2008, 372(9634): 201.

66. Dwan K, Gamble C, Williamson PR, Kirkham JJ, Reporting Bias G. Systematic review of the empirical evidence of study publication bias and outcome reporting bias - an updated review. PLoS One, 2013, 8(7): e66844.

67. University of York. PROSPERO, an international database of prospectively registered systematic reviews in health and social care. 2011, PROSPERO was launched by the NIHR on 22 February 2011 at U of York's Centre for Reviews and Dissemination. http://www.crd.york.ac.uk/prospero/search.asp.

68. Riley RD, Lambert PC, Staessen JA, Wang J, Gueyffier F, Thijs L, Boutitie F. Meta-analysis of continuous outcomes combining individual patient data and aggregate data. Stat Med, 2008, 27(11): 1870-1893.

69. Riley RD, Steyerberg EW. Meta-analysis of a binary outcome using individual participant data and aggregate data. Res Synth Methods, 2010, 1(1): 2-19.

70. Light RJ, Pillemer DB. Summing up: The science of reviewing research. 1984, Cambridge, MA: Harvard University Press.

71. Greenland S, Lanes S, Jara M. Estimating effects from randomized trials with discontinuations: the need for intent-to-treat design and G-estimation. Clin Trials, 2008, 5(1): 5-13.

72. Toh S, Hernan MA. Causal inference from longitudinal studies with baseline randomization. Int J Biostat, 2008, 4(1): Article 22.

73. Toh S, Hernandez-Diaz S, Logan R, Robins JM, Hernan MA. Estimating absolute risks in the presence of nonadherence: an application to a follow-up study with baseline randomization. Epidemiology, 2010, 21(4): 528-539.

74. Hernan MA, Hernandez-Diaz S. Beyond the intention-to-treat in comparative effectiveness research. Clin Trials, 2012, 9(1): 48-55.

75. Montedori A, Bonacini MI, Casazza G, Luchetta ML, Duca P, Cozzolino F, Abraha I. Modified versus standard intention-to-treat reporting: are there differences in methodological quality, sponsorship, and findings in randomized trials? A cross-sectional study. Trials, 2011, 12: 58.

76. Lewis JA, Machin D. Intention to treat-who should use ITT? Br J Cancer, 1993, 68(4): 647-650.

77. Cooper AJ, Lettis S, Chapman CL, Evans SJ, Waller PC, Shakir S, Payvandi N, Murray AB. Developing tools for the safety specification in risk management plans: lessons learned from a pilot project. Pharmacoepidemiol Drug Saf, 2008, 17(5): 445-454.

78. O'Neill RT. Assessment of safety. in Biopharmaceutical Statistics for Drug Development. 1988, Marcel Dekker.

79. Proschan MA, Lan KK, Wittes JT. Statistical Methods for Monitoring Clinical Trials. 2006, New York: Springer.

80. MedDRA Home Page. Medical Dictionary for Regulatory Activities. MedDRA MSSO (Medical Dictionary for Regulatory Activities Maintenance and Support Services Organization), 2015, 2013. http://www.meddra.org/.

81. U.S. Food and Drug Administration. Guidance for Industry: Suicidal Ideation and Behavior: Prospective Assessment of Occurrence in Clinical Trials, August 2012, accessed at. 2012. http://www.fda.gov/drugs/guidancecomplianceregulatoryinformation/guidances/ucm315156.htm.

82. Posner K, Oquendo MA, Gould M, Stanley B, Davies M. Columbia Classification Algorithm of Suicide Assessment (C-CASA): classification of suicidal events in the FDA's pediatric suicidal risk analysis of antidepressants. Am J Psychiatry, 2007, 164(7): 1035-1043.

83. Golder S, McIntosh HM, Loke Y. Identifying systematic reviews of the adverse effects of health care interventions. BMC Med Res Methodol, 2006, 6: 22.

84. Sherman RB, Woodcock J, Norden J, Grandinetti C, Temple RJ. New FDA regulation to improve safety reporting in clinical trials. N Engl J Med, 2011, 365(1): 3-5.

85. ICH International Conference on Harmonisation. ICH E3 Guideline: Structure and Content of Clinical Study Reports. 1995. http://www.ich.org/fileadmin/Public_Web_Site/ICH_Products/Guidelines/Efficacy/E3/E3_Guideline.pdf.

86. Huang HY, Andrews E, Jones J, Skovron ML, Tilson H. Pitfalls in meta-analyses on adverse events reported from clinical trials. Pharmacoepidemiol Drug Saf, 2011, 20(10): 1014-1020.

87. Loke YK, Price D, Herxheimer A, Group CAEM. Systematic reviews of adverse effects: framework for a structured approach. BMC Med Res Methodol, 2007, 7: 32.

88. ICH International Conference on Harmonisation. ICH M4E Guideline on Enhancing the Format and Structure of Benefit-Risk Information in ICH. 2014. http://www.ich.org/products/ctd/ctdsingle/article/revision-of-m4e-guideline-on-enhancing-the-format-and-structure-of-benefit-risk-information-in-ich.html.

89. U.S. Food and Drug Administration. Guidance for Industry: Premarketing Risk Assessment. 2012. http://www.fda.gov/downloads/RegulatoryInformation/Guidances/UCM126958.pdf.

90. Egger M, Zellweger-Zahner T, Schneider M, Junker C, Lengeler C, Antes G. Language bias in randomised controlled trials published in English and German. Lancet, 1997, 350(9074): 326-329.

91. Institute of Medicine. Finding What Works in Health Care: Standards for Systematic Reviews. 2011, Washington, DC: The National Academies Press.

92. Jones AP, Remmington T, Williamson PR, Ashby D, Smyth RL. High prevalence but low impact of data extraction and reporting errors were found in Cochrane systematic reviews. J Clin Epidemiol, 2005, 58(7): 741-742.

93. Horton J, Vandermeer B, Hartling L, Tjosvold L, Klassen TP, Buscemi N. Systematic review data extraction: cross-sectional study showed that experience did not increase accuracy. J Clin Epidemiol, 2010, 63(3): 289-298.

94. Buscemi N, Hartling L, Vandermeer B, Tjosvold L, Klassen TP. Single data extraction generated more errors than double data extraction in systematic reviews. J Clin Epidemiol, 2006, 59(7): 697-703.

95. Centre for Reviews and Dissemination. Systematic reviews: CRD's guidance for undertaking reviews in health care. 2009. www.york.ac.uk/media/crd/Systematic_Reviews.pdf.

96. Ware JH, Vetrovec GW, Miller AB, Van Tosh A, Gaffney M, Yunis C, Arteaga C, Borer JS. Cardiovascular safety of varenicline: patient-level meta-analysis of randomized, blinded, placebo-controlled trials. Am J Ther, 2013, 20(3): 235-246.

97. Shuster JJ. Empirical vs natural weighting in random effects meta-analysis. Stat Med, 2010, 29(12): 1259-1265.

98. Berlin JA, Kim C. The use of meta-analysis in pharmacoepidemiology. in Pharmacoepidemiology, Fourth, S.B. (ed), Editor. 2005, John Wiley and Sons: Chichester. 681-707.

99. Colditz GA, Berkey CS, Mosteller F, Brewer TF, Wilson ME, Burdick E, Fineberg HV. The efficacy of bacillus Calmette-Guerin vaccination of newborns and infants in the prevention of tuberculosis: meta-analyses of the published literature. Pediatrics, 1995, 96(1 Pt 1): 29-35.

100. Colditz GA, Brewer TF, Berkey CS, Wilson ME, Burdick E, Fineberg HV, Mosteller F. Efficacy of BCG vaccine in the prevention of tuberculosis. Meta-analysis of the published literature. JAMA, 1994, 271(9): 698-702.

101. Furukawa TA, Streiner DL, Hori S. Discrepancies among megatrials. J Clin Epidemiol, 2000, 53(12): 1193-1199.

102. LeLorier J, Grégoire G, Benhaddad A, Lapierre J, Derderian F. Discrepancies between meta-analyses and subsequent large randomized, controlled trials. N Engl J Med, 1997, 337(8): 536-542.

103. U.S. Food and Drug Administration. Statistical review and evaluation antiepileptic drugs and suicidality. 2008, 45. http://www.fda.gov/Drugs/DrugSafety/PostmarketDrugSafetyInformationforPatientsandProviders/DrugSafetyInformationforHeathcareProfessionals/ucm070651.htm.

104. Senn SJ. Overstating the evidence: double counting in meta-analysis and related problems. BMC Med Res Methodol, 2009, 9(10).

105. Thompson SG, Higgins JP. How should meta-regression analyses be undertaken and interpreted? Stat Med, 2002, 21(11): 1559-1573.

106. Gleser LJ, Olkin I. Stochastically dependent effect sizes. in The handbook of research synthesis and meta-analysis, 2nd, H. Cooper, L.V. Hedges, and J.C. Valentine, Editors. 1994, Russell Sage Foundation: New York.

107. Berlin JA, Colditz GA. The role of meta-analysis in the regulatory process for foods, drugs, and devices. JAMA, 1999, 281(9): 830-834.

108. Temple R. Meta-analysis and epidemiologic studies in drug development and postmarketing surveillance. JAMA, 1999, 281(9): 841-844.

109. Hernandez AV, Walker E, Ioannidis JP, Kattan MW. Challenges in meta-analysis of randomized clinical trials for rare harmful cardiovascular events: the case of rosiglitazone. Am Heart J, 2008, 156(1): 23-30.

110. Feinstein AR. Meta-analysis: statistical alchemy for the 21st century. J Clin Epidemiol, 1995, 48(1): 71-79.

111. Chalmers TC. Problems induced by meta-analyses. Stat Med, 1991, 10(6): 971-979; discussion 979-980.

112. Moher D, Jadad AR, Nichol G, Penman M, Tugwell P, Walsh S. Assessing the quality of randomized controlled trials: an annotated bibliography of scales and checklists. Control Clin Trials, 1995, 16(1): 62-73.

113. Chalmers TC, Smith H, Blackburn B, Silverman B, Schroeder B, Reitman D, Ambroz A. A method for assessing the quality of a randomized control trial. Control Clin Trials, 1981, 2(1): 31-49.

114. Olivo SA, Macedo LG, Gadotti IC, Fuentes J, Stanton T, Magee DJ. Scales to assess the quality of randomized controlled trials: a systematic review. Phys Ther, 2008, 88(2): 156-175.

115. Juni P, Altman DG, Egger M. Systematic reviews in health care: Assessing the quality of controlled clinical trials. BMJ, 2001, 323(7303): 42-46.

116. Borghouts JA, Koes BW, Bouter LM. The clinical course and prognostic factors of non-specific neck pain: a systematic review. Pain, 1998, 77(1): 1-13.

117. Greenland S. Quality scores are useless and potentially misleading: reply to "Re: A critical look at some popular analytic methods". Am J Epidemiol, 1994, 140(3): 300-301.

118. Fabricatore AN, Wadden TA, Moore RH, Butryn ML, Gravallese EA, Erondu NE, Heymsfield SB, Nguyen AM. Attrition from randomized controlled trials of pharmacological weight loss agents: a systematic review and analysis. Obes Rev, 2009, 10(3): 333-341.

119. Rosenbaum PR, Rubin DB. Assessing sensitivity to an unobserved binary covariate in an observational study with binary outcome. J R Stat Soc, 1983: 212-218.

120. Lin DY, Psaty BM, Kronmal RA. Assessing the sensitivity of regression results to unmeasured confounders in observational studies. Biometrics, 1998, 54(3): 948-963.

121. Schneeweiss S, Glynn RJ, Tsai EH, Avorn J, Solomon DH. Adjusting for unmeasured confounders in pharmacoepidemiologic claims data using external information: the example of COX2 inhibitors and myocardial infarction. Epidemiology, 2005, 16(1): 17-24.

122. Sturmer T, Schneeweiss S, Avorn J, Glynn RJ. Adjusting effect estimates for unmeasured confounding with validation data using propensity score calibration. Am J Epidemiol, 2005, 162(3): 279-289.

123. Kesten S, Plautz M, Piquette CA, Habib MP, Niewoehner DE. Premature discontinuation of patients: a potential bias in COPD clinical trials. Eur Respir J, 2007, 30(5): 898-906.

124. Montgomery SA, Baldwin DS, Riley A. Antidepressant medications: a review of the evidence for drug-induced sexual dysfunction. J Affect Disord, 2002, 69(1-3): 119-140.

125. Garbe E, Suissa S. Hormone replacement therapy and acute coronary outcomes: methodological issues between randomized and observational studies. Hum Reprod, 2004, 19(1): 8-13.

126. Ioannidis JP, Lau J. Completeness of safety reporting in randomized trials: an evaluation of 7 medical areas. JAMA, 2001, 285(4): 437-443.

127. Pitrou I, Boutron I, Ahmad N, Ravaud P. Reporting of safety results in published reports of randomized controlled trials. Arch Intern Med, 2009, 169(19): 1756-1761.

128. Michele TM, Pinheiro S, Iyasu S. The safety of tiotropium-the FDA's conclusions. N Engl J Med, 2010, 363(12): 1097-1099.

129. Mallinckrodt C, Chuang-Stein C, McSorley P, Schwartz J, Archibald DG, Perahia DG, Detke MJ, Alphs L. A case study comparing a randomized withdrawal trial and a double-blind long-term trial for assessing the long-term efficacy of an antidepressant. Pharm Stat, 2007, 6(1): 9-22.

130. Perahia DG, Maina G, Thase ME, Spann ME, Wang F, Walker DJ, Detke MJ. Duloxetine in the prevention of depressive recurrences: a randomized, double-blind, placebo-controlled trial. J Clin Psychiatry, 2009, 70(5): 706-716.

131. Ghaemi SN. The failure to know what isn't known: negative publication bias with lamotrigine and a glimpse inside peer review. Evid Based Ment Health, 2009, 12(3): 65-68.

132. Egger M, Davey Smith G, Schneider M, Minder C. Bias in meta-analysis detected by a simple, graphical test. BMJ, 1997, 315(7109): 629-634.

133. Sterne JA, Harbord RM. Funnel plots in meta-analysis. Stata Journal, 2004, 4: 127-141.

134. U.S. National Institutes for Health. ClinicalTrials.gov. 2007, ClinicalTrials.gov is a registry and results database of publicly and privately supported clinical studies of human participants conducted around the world. https://clinicaltrials.gov/.

135. Yahav D, Paul M, Fraser A, Sarid N, Leibovici L. Efficacy and safety of cefepime: a systematic review and meta-analysis. Lancet Infect Dis, 2007, 7(5): 338-348.

136. Brocklebank D, Wright J, Cates C. Systematic review of clinical effectiveness of pressurised metered dose inhalers versus other hand held inhaler devices for delivering corticosteroids in asthma. BMJ, 2001, 323(7318): 896-900.

137. Olkin I, Sampson A. Comparison of meta-analysis versus analysis of variance of individual patient data. Biometrics, 1998, 54(1): 317-322.

138. Szczech LA, Berlin JA, Feldman HI. The effect of antilymphocyte induction therapy on renal allograft survival. A meta-analysis of individual patient-level data. Anti-Lymphocyte Antibody Induction Therapy Study Group. Ann Intern Med, 1998, 128(10): 817-826.

139. Berlin JA, Santanna J, Schmid CH, Szczech LA, Feldman HI, Anti-Lymphocyte Antibody Induction Therapy Study G. Individual patient- versus group-level data meta-regressions for the investigation of treatment effect modifiers: ecological bias rears its ugly head. Stat Med, 2002, 21(3): 371-387.

140. Lambert PC, Sutton AJ, Abrams KR, Jones DR. A comparison of summary patient-level covariates in meta-regression with individual patient data meta-analysis. J Clin Epidemiol, 2002, 55(1): 86-94.

141. Schmid CH, Stark PC, Berlin JA, Landais P, Lau J. Meta-regression detected associations between heterogeneous treatment effects and study-level, but not patient-level, factors. J Clin Epidemiol, 2004, 57(7): 683-697.

142. Vandenbroucke JP. What is the best evidence for determining harms of medical treatment? CMAJ, 2006, 174(5): 645-646.

143. Gagne JJ, Schneeweiss S. Comment on ‚empirical assessment of methods for risk identification in healthcare data: results from the experiments of the Observational Medical Outcomes Partnership'. Stat Med, 2013, 32(6): 1073-1074.

144. Rothman K, Greenland S, Lash T. Modern Epidemiology. 3rd Edition ed. 2008, Philadelphia, PA: Lippincott, Williams & Wilkins.

145. Strom BL. Study Designs Available for Pharmacoepidemiology Studies. in Pharmacoepidemiology, Fourth (4th). 2006, John Wiley & Sons.

146. Pearce N. Classification of epidemiological study designs. Int J Epidemiol, 2012, 41(2): 393-7.

147. Loke YK, Golder SP, Vandenbroucke JP. Comprehensive evaluations of the adverse effects of drugs: importance of appropriate study selection and data sources. Ther Adv Drug Saf, 2011, 2(2): 59-68.

148. Golder S, Loke YK, Bland M. Meta-analyses of adverse effects data derived from randomised controlled trials as compared to observational studies: methodological overview. PLoS Med, 2011, 8(5): e1001026.

149. Papanikolaou PN, Christidi GD, Ioannidis JP. Comparison of evidence on harms of medical interventions in randomized and nonrandomized studies. CMAJ, 2006, 174(5): 635-641.

150. Neyarapally GA, Hammad TA, Pinheiro SP, Iyasu S. Review of quality assessment tools for the evaluation of pharmacoepidemiological safety studies. BMJ open, 2012, 2(5).

151. ENCePP. European Network of Centres for Pharmacoepidemiology and Pharmacovigilance. 2006. http://www.encepp.eu/encepp/studiesDatabase.jsp.

152. Chavers S, Fife D, Wacholtz M, Stang P, Berlin J. Registration of Observational Studies: perspectives from an industry-based epidemiology group. Pharmacoepidemiol Drug Saf, 2011, 20(10): 1009-1013.

153. von Elm E, Altman DG, Egger M, Pocock SJ, Gøtzsche PC, Vandenbroucke JP, Initiative S. The Strengthening the Reporting of Observational Studies in Epidemiology (STROBE) statement: guidelines for reporting observational studies. Epidemiology, 2007, 18(6): 800-804.

154. Collaborative Group on Hormonal Factors in Breast Cancer. Breast cancer and hormone replacement therapy: collaborative reanalysis of data from 51 epidemiological studies of 52,705 women with breast cancer and 108,411 women without breast cancer. Collaborative Group on Hormonal Factors in Breast Cancer. Lancet, 1997, 350(9084): 1047-1059.

155. Salanti G, Dias S, Welton NJ, Ades AE, Golfinopoulos V, Kyrgiou M, Mauri D, Ioannidis JP. Evaluating novel agent effects in multiple-treatments meta-regression. Stat Med, 2010, 29(23): 2369-2383.

156. Bucher HC, Guyatt GH, Griffith LE, Walter SD. The results of direct and indirect treatment comparisons in meta-analysis of randomized controlled trials. J Clin Epidemiol, 1997, 50(6): 683-691.

157. Lumley T. Network meta-analysis for indirect treatment comparisons. Stat Med, 2002, 21(16): 2313-2324.

158. Lu G, Ades A. Assessing evidence inconsistency in mixed treatment comparisons. Journal of the American Statistical Association, 2006, 101(474).

159. Higgins JPT, Jackson D, Barrett JK, Lu G, Ades AE, White IR. Consistency and inconsistency in network meta-analysis: concepts and models for multi-arm studies. Res Synth Methods, 2012, 3(2): 98-110.

160. Donegan S, Williamson P, D'Alessandro U, Tudur Smith C. Assessing key assumptions of network meta-analysis: a review of methods. Res Synth Methods, 2013, 4(4): 291-323.

161. Coxib and traditional NSAID Trialists' (CNT) Collaboration, Bhala N, Emberson J, Merhi A, Abramson S, Arber N, Baron JA, et al. Vascular and upper gastrointestinal effects of non-steroidal anti-inflammatory drugs: meta-analyses of individual participant data from randomised trials. Lancet, 2013, 382(9894): 769-779.

162. Mills EJ, Thorlund K, Ioannidis JP. Demystifying trial networks and network meta-analysis. BMJ, 2013, 346: f2914.

163. Deeks JJ, Altman DG. Effect measure for meta-analysis of trials with binary outcomes. in Systematic reviews in health care: Meta-analysis in context, 2nd, M. Egger, G.D. Smith, and D.G. Altman, Editors. 2008, BMJ Publishing: London, UK.

164. Sutton AJ, Cooper NJ, Lambert PC, Jones DR, Abrams KR, Sweeting MJ. Meta-analysis of rare and adverse event data. Expert Rev Pharmacoecon Outcomes Res, 2002, 2(4): 367-379.

165. Deeks JJ. Issues in the selection of a summary statistic for meta-analysis of clinical trials with binary outcomes. Stat Med, 2002, 21(11): 1575-600.

166. Engels EA, Schmid CH, Terrin N, Olkin I, Lau J. Heterogeneity and statistical significance in meta-analysis: an empirical study of 125 meta-analyses. Stat Med, 2000, 19(13): 1707-1728.

167. Localio AR, Margolis DJ, Berlin JA. Relative risks and confidence intervals were easily computed indirectly from multivariable logistic regression. J Clin Epidemiol, 2007, 60: 874-882.

168. Grieve AP. The number needed to treat: a useful clinical measure or a case of the Emperor's new clothes? Pharm Stat, 2003, 2(2): 87-102.

169. Smeeth L, Haines A, Ebrahim S. Numbers needed to treat derived from meta-analyses–sometimes informative, usually misleading. BMJ, 1999, 318(7197): 1548-1551.

170. Parmar MK, Torri V, Stewart L. Extracting summary statistics to perform meta-analyses of the published literature for survival endpoints. Stat Med, 1998, 17(24): 2815-2834.

171. Williamson PR, Smith CT, Hutton JL, Marson AG. Aggregate data meta-analysis with time-to-event outcomes. Stat Med, 2002, 21(22): 3337-3351.

172. Moodie PF, Nelson NA, Koch GG. A non-parametric procedure for evaluating treatment effect in the meta-analysis of survival data. Stat Med, 2004, 23(7): 1075-1093.

173. Sutton AJ, Abrams KR, Jones DR, Jones DR, Sheldon TA, Song F. Methods for meta-analysis in medical research. 2000, Chichester, UK: J. Wiley.

174. Simmonds MC, Higgins JP, Stewart LA, Tierney JF, Clarke MJ, Thompson SG. Meta-analysis of individual patient data from randomized trials: a review of methods used in practice. Clin Trials, 2005, 2(3): 209-217.

175. Hedges LV, Olkin I. Statistical methods for meta-analysis. 1985, Orlando, FL: Academic Press.

176. Sweeting MJ, Sutton AJ, Lambert PC. Correction. Stat Med, 2006, 25: 2700.

177. Sweeting MJ, Sutton AJ, Lambert PC. What to add to nothing? Use and avoidance of continuity corrections in meta-analysis of sparse data. Stat Med, 2004, 23(9): 1351-1375.

178. Bennett MM, Crowe BJ, Price KL, Stamey JD, Seaman JW, Jr. Comparison of bayesian and frequentist meta-analytical approaches for analyzing time to event data. J Biopharm Stat, 2013, 23(1): 129-145.

179. Bradburn MJ, Deeks JJ, Berlin JA, Russell Localio A. Much ado about nothing: a comparison of the performance of meta-analytical methods with rare events. Stat Med, 2007, 26(1): 53-77.

180. Tian L, Cai T, Pfeffer MA, Piankov N, Cremieux PY, Wei LJ. Exact and efficient inference procedure for meta-analysis and its application to the analysis of independent 2 x 2 tables with all available data but without artificial continuity correction. Biostatistics, 2009, 10(2): 275-281.

181. Rucker G, Schwarzer G, Carpenter JR, Binder H, Schumacher M. Treatment-effect estimates adjusted for small-study effects via a limit meta-analysis. Biostatistics, 2011, 12(1): 122-142.

182. Yusuf S, Peto R, Lewis J, Collins R, Sleight P. Beta blockade during and after myocardial infarction: an overview of the randomized trials. Prog Cardiovasc Dis, 1985, 27(5): 335-71.

183. Greenland S, Salvan A. Bias in the one-step method for pooling study results. Stat Med, 1990, 9(3): 247-252.

184. Cai T, Parast L, Ryan L. Meta-analysis for rare events. Stat Med, 2010, 29(20): 2078-2089.

185. Firth D. Bias reduction of maximum likelihood estimates. Biometrika, 1993, 80(1): 27-38.

186. Heinze G, Schemper M. A solution to the problem of monotone likelihood in Cox regression. Biometrics, 2001, 57(1): 114-119.

187. The Handbook of Research Synthesis and Meta-analysis. 2nd ed. 2009, Russell Sage Foundation: New York, New York. 615.

188. Bailey KR. Inter-study differences: How should they influence the interpretation and analysis of results? Stat Med, 1987, 6(3): 351-358.

189. Peto R. Why do we need systematic overviews of randomized trials? Stat Med, 1987, 6(3): 233-244.

190. Poole C, Greenland S. Random-effects meta-analyses are not always conservative. Am J Epidemiol, 1999, 150(5): 469-475.

191. Berlin JA, Crowe BJ, Whalen E, Xia HA, Koro CE, Kuebler J. Meta-analysis of clinical trial safety data in a drug development program: answers to frequently asked questions. Clin Trials, 2013, 10(1): 20-31.

192. FDA. Reviewer Guidance: Conducting a Clinical Safety Review on a New Product Application and Preparing a Report on the Review. 2005. http://www.fda.gov/downloads/Drugs/GuidanceComplianceRegulatoryInformation/Guidances/ucm072974.pdf.

193. DerSimonian R, Laird N. Meta-analysis in clinical trials. Control Clin Trials, 1986, 7(3): 177-188.

194. Jackson D, Bowden J, Baker R. How does the DerSimonian and Laird procedure for random effects meta-analysis compare with its more efficient but harder to compute counterparts? J Stat Plan Inference, 2010, 140(4): 961-970.

195. Cornell JE, Mulrow CD, Localio R, Stack CB, Meibohm AR, Guallar E, Goodman SN. Random-effects meta-analysis of inconsistent effects: a time for change. Ann Intern Med, 2014, 160(4): 267-270.

196. IntHout J, Ioannidis JP, Borm GF. The Hartung-Knapp-Sidik-Jonkman method for random effects meta-analysis is straightforward and considerably outperforms the standard DerSimonian-Laird method. BMC Med Res Methodol, 2014, 14: 25.

197. Cochran W, Cox G. Experimental Designs. 2nd ed. 1992, New York: Wiley.

198. Higgins JP, Thompson SG. Quantifying heterogeneity in a meta-analysis. Stat Med, 2002, 21(11): 1539-1558.

199. Sutton AJ, Abrams KR. Bayesian methods in meta-analysis and evidence synthesis. Stat Methods Med Res, 2001, 10(4): 277-303.

200. Bayes TR. An essay towards solving a problem in the doctrine of chances. Philosophical transactions of the royal society of London, 1763: 370-418.

201. McGrayne SB. The Theory That Would Not Die: How Bayes' Rule Cracked The Enigma Code, Hunted Down Russian Submarines, & Emerged Triumphant from Two Centuries of Controversy. 2011, New Haven & London: Yale University Press.

202. Warn D, Thompson S, Spiegelhalter D. Bayesian random effects meta-analysis of trials with binary outcomes: methods for the absolute risk difference and relative risk scales. Stat Med, 2002, 21(11): 1601-1623.

203. Higgins JPT, Thompson SG, Spiegelhalter DJ. A re-evaluation of random-effects meta-analysis. J R Stat Soc Ser A Stat Soc, 2009, 172(1): 137-159.

204. Lambert PC, Sutton AJ, Burton PR, Abrams KR, Jones DR. How vague is vague? A simulation study of the impact of the use of vague prior distributions in MCMC using WinBUGS. Stat Med, 2005, 24(15): 2401-2428.

205. Lee KJ, Thompson SG. Flexible parametric models for random-effects distributions. Stat Med, 2008, 27(3): 418-434.

206. Muthukumarana S, Tiwari RC. Meta-analysis using Dirichlet process. Stat Methods Med Res, 2012.

207. Mesgarpour B, Heidinger BH, Schwameis M, Kienbacher C, Walsh C, Schmitz S, Herkner H. Safety of off-label erythropoiesis stimulating agents in critically ill patients: a meta-analysis. Intensive Care Med, 2013, 39(11): 1896-1908.

208. Ohlssen D, Price KL, Xia HA, Hong H, Kerman J, Fu H, Quartey G, Heilmann CR, Ma H, Carlin BP. Guidance on the implementation and reporting of a drug safety Bayesian network meta-analysis. Pharm Stat, 2014, 13(1): 55-70.

209. Higgins JP, Spiegelhalter DJ. Being sceptical about meta-analyses: a Bayesian perspective on magnesium trials in myocardial infarction. Int J Epidemiol, 2002, 31(1): 96-104.

210. Askling J, Fahrbach K, Nordstrom B, Ross S, Schmid CH, Symmons D. Cancer risk with tumor necrosis factor alpha (TNF) inhibitors: meta-analysis of randomized controlled trials of adalimumab, etanercept, and infliximab using patient level data. Pharmacoepidemiol Drug Saf, 2011, 20(2): 119-130.

211. Kaizar EE, Greenhouse JB, Seltman H, Kelleher K. Do antidepressants cause suicidality in children? A Bayesian meta-analysis. Clin Trials, 2006, 3(2): 73-98.

212. Ibrahim JG, Chen MH, Xia HA, Liu T. Bayesian meta-experimental design: evaluating cardiovascular risk in new antidiabetic therapies to treat type 2 diabetes. Biometrics, 2012, 68(2): 578-586.

213. Hedges LV, Pigott TD. The power of statistical tests for moderators in meta-analysis. Psychol Methods, 2004, 9(4): 426-445.

214. Hedges LV, Pigott TD. The power of statistical tests in meta-analysis. Psychol Methods, 2001, 6(3): 203-217.

215. Hemminki E. Study of information submitted by drug companies to licensing authorities. BMJ, 1980, 280(6217): 833-836.

216. Easterbrook PJ, Berlin JA, Gopalan R, Matthews DR. Publication bias in clinical research. Lancet, 1991, 337(8746): 867-872.

217. Gotzsche PC. Reference bias in reports of drug trials. BMJ (Clin Res Ed), 1987, 295(6599): 654-656.

218. Gotzsche PC. Multiple publication of reports of drug trials. Eur J Clin Pharmacol, 1989, 36(5): 429-432.

219. Pocock SJ, Hughes MD, Lee RJ. Statistical problems in the reporting of clinical trials. A survey of three medical journals. N Engl J Med, 1987, 317(7): 426-432.

220. Tannock IF. False-positive results in clinical trials: multiple significance tests and the problem of unreported comparisons. J Natl Cancer Inst, 1996, 88(3-4): 206-207.

221. Heres S, Davis J, Maino K, Jetzinger E, Kissling W, Leucht S. Why olanzapine beats risperidone, risperidone beats quetiapine, and quetiapine beats olanzapine: an exploratory analysis of head-to-head comparison studies of second-generation antipsychotics. Am J Psychiatry, 2006, 163(2): 185-194.

222. Melander H, Ahlqvist-Rastad J, Meijer G, Beermann B. Evidence b(i)ased medicine—selective reporting from studies sponsored by pharmaceutical industry: review of studies in new drug applications. BMJ, 2003, 326(7400): 1171-1173.

223. Little RJ, Rubin DB. Statistical Analysis with Missing Data. 2002, Oxford, England: Wiley-Interscience.

224. National Institute for Health and Care Excellence (NICE). Guide to the Methods of Technology Appraisal. 2013. http://www.nice.org.uk/article/pmg9/chapter/Foreword.

225. National Institute for Health and Care Excellence (NICE). The guidelines manual. 2012. http://publications.nice.org.uk/the guidelines manual pmg6.

226. Turner NL, Dias S, Ades AE, Welton NJ. A Bayesian framework to account for uncertainty due to missing binary outcome data in pairwise meta-analysis. Stat Med, 2015, 34(12): 2062-2080.

227. Higgins JP, White IR, Wood AM. Imputation methods for missing outcome data in meta-analysis of clinical trials. Clin Trials, 2008, 5(3): 225-239.

228. Biester K, Lange S. The multiplicity problem in systematic reviews. XIII Cochrane Colloquium. 2005, Melbourne, Australia. 153.

229. Baum ML, Anish DS, Chalmers TC, Sacks HS, Smith H, Jr., Fagerstrom RM. A survey of clinical trials of antibiotic prophylaxis in colon surgery: evidence against further use of no-treatment controls. N Engl J Med, 1981, 305(14): 795-799.

230. Lau J, Antman EM, Jimenez-Silva J, Kupelnick B, Mosteller F, Chalmers TC. Cumulative meta-analysis of therapeutic trials for myocardial infarction. N Engl J Med, 1992, 327(4): 248-254.

231. Flather MD, Farkouh ME, Pogue JM, Yusuf S. Strengths and limitations of meta-analysis: larger studies may be more reliable. Control Clin Trials, 1997, 18(6): 568-579; discussion 661-666.

232. Whitehead A. A prospectively planned cumulative meta-analysis applied to a series of concurrent clinical trials. Stat Med, 1997, 16(24): 2901-2913.

233. Pogue JM, Yusuf S. Cumulating evidence from randomized trials: utilizing sequential monitoring boundaries for cumulative meta-analysis. Control Clin Trials, 1997, 18(6): 580-93; discussion 661-666.

234. van der Tweel I, Bollen C. Sequential meta-analysis: an efficient decision-making tool. Clin Trials, 2010, 7(2): 136-146.

235. O'Brien PC, Fleming TR. A multiple testing procedure for clinical trials. Biometrics, 1979, 35(3): 549-556.

236. Lan KK, DeMets DL. Discrete sequential boundaries for clinical trials. Biometrika, 1983, 70(3): 659-663.

237. Kulinskaya E, Wood J. Trial sequential methods for meta-analysis. Res Synth Methods, 2014, 5(3): 212-220.

238. Imberger G, Wetterslev J, Gluud C. Trial sequential analysis has the potential to improve the reliability of conclusions in meta-analysis. Contemp Clin Trials, 2013, 36(1): 254-255.

239. Miladinovic B, Mhaskar R, Hozo I, Kumar A, Mahony H, Djulbegovic B. Optimal information size in trial sequential analysis of time-to-event outcomes reveals potentially inconclusive results because of the risk of random error. J Clin Epidemiol, 2013, 66(6): 654-659.

240. Higgins JPT, Whitehead A, Simmonds M. Sequential methods for random-effects meta-analysis. Stat Med, 2011, 30(9): 903-921.

241. Thorlund K, Devereaux PJ, Wetterslev J, Guyatt G, Ioannidis JP, Thabane L, Gluud LL, Als-Nielsen B, Gluud C. Can trial sequential monitoring boundaries reduce spurious inferences from meta-analyses? Int J Epidemiol, 2009, 38(1): 276-286.

242. Brok J, Thorlund K, Gluud C, Wetterslev J. Trial sequential analysis reveals insufficient information size and potentially false positive results in many meta-analyses. J Clin Epidemiol, 2008, 61(8): 763-769.

243. Wetterslev J, Thorlund K, Brok J, Gluud C. Trial sequential analysis may establish when firm evidence is reached in cumulative meta-analysis. J Clin Epidemiol, 2008, 61(1): 64-75.

244. Jennison C, Turnbull BW. Meta-analyses and adaptive group sequential designs in the clinical development process. J Biopharm Stat, 2005, 15(4): 537-558.

245. Quan H, Ma Y, Zheng Y, Cho M, Lorenzato C, Hecquet C. Adaptive and repeated cumulative meta-analyses for safety signal detection during a new drug development process. Statistical Technical Report #54 (Sanofi), 2011, 54.

246. Lan KK, Hu M, Cappelleri JC. Applying the law of iterated logarithm to cumulative meta-analysis of a continuous endpoint. Statistica Sinica (Pfizer Inc.), 2003, 13: 1135-1145.

247. Hu M, Cappelleri JC, Lan KK. Applying the law of iterated logarithm to control type I error in cumulative meta-analysis of binary outcomes. Clin Trials, 2007, 4(4): 329-340.

248. Lau J, Schmid CH, Chalmers TC. Cumulative meta-analysis of clinical trials builds evidence for exemplary medical care. J Clin Epidemiol, 1995, 48(1): 45-57; discussion 59-60.

249. Chen MH, Ibrahim JG, Amy Xia HA, Liu T, Hennessey V. Bayesian sequential meta-analysis design in evaluating cardiovascular risk in a new antidiabetic drug development program. Stat Med, 2014, 33(9): 1600-1618.

250. Jeffreys H. An invariant form for the prior probability in estimation problems,. in Royal Statistical Society of London. 1946. London.

251. Bender R, Bunce C, Clarke M, Gates S, Lange S, Pace NL, Thorlund K. Attention should be given to multiplicity issues in systematic reviews. J Clin Epidemiol, 2008, 61(9): 857-865.

252. Thompson SG. Why sources of heterogeneity in meta-analysis should be investigated. BMJ, 1994, 309(6965): 1351-1355.

253. U.S. Food and Drug Administration. Guidance for industry non-inferiority clinical trials. US Department of Health and Human Services and US Food and Drug Administration, Washington, DC, 2010. http://download.bioon.com.cn/upload/201305/19233453_9245.pdf.

254. Deeks JJ, Altman DG, Bradburn MJ. Statistical methods for examining heterogeneity and combining results from several studies in meta-analysis. in Systematic Reviews in Health Care: Meta-analysis in context, 2nd edition, M. Egger, G.D. Smith, and D.G. Altman, Editors. 2001, BMJ Publishing Group: London.

255. Thompson SG, Sharp SJ. Explaining heterogeneity in meta-analysis: a comparison of methods. Stat Med, 1999, 18(20): 2693-2708.

256. Gagnier JJ, Moher D, Boon H, Bombardier C, Beyene J. An empirical study using permutation-based resampling in meta-regression. Syst Rev, 2012, 1: 18.

257. Morgenstern H. Uses of ecologic analysis in epidemiologic research. Am J Public Health, 1982, 72(12): 1336-1344.

258. Greenland S. Quantitative methods in the review of epidemiologic literature. Epidemiol Rev, 1987, 9: 1-30.

259. Oxman AD, Guyatt GH. A consumer's guide to subgroup analyses. Ann Intern Med, 1992, 116(1): 78-84.

260. Yusuf S, Wittes J, Probstfield J, Tyroler HA. Analysis and interpretation of treatment effects in subgroups of patients in randomized clinical trials. JAMA, 1991, 266(1): 93-98.

261. Rothwell PM. External validity of randomised controlled trials: "to whom do the results of this trial apply?". Lancet, 2005, 365(9453): 82-93.

262. Olkin I. Re: "A critical look at some popular meta-analytic methods". Am J Epidemiol, 1994, 140(3): 297-299; discussion 300-301.

263. Egger M, Smith GD, Sterne JA. Uses and abuses of meta-analysis. Clin Med, 2001, 1(6): 478-484.

264. Lewis S, Clarke M. Forest plots: trying to see the wood and the trees. BMJ, 2001, 322(7300): 1479-1480.

265. Stroup DF, Berlin JA, Morton SC, Olkin I, Williamson GD, Rennie D, Moher D, Becker BJ, Sipe TA, Thacker SB. Meta-analysis of observational studies in epidemiology: a proposal for reporting. Meta-analysis Of Observational Studies in Epidemiology (MOOSE) group. JAMA, 2000, 283(15): 2008-2012.

266. Liberati A, Altman DG, Tetzlaff J, Mulrow C, Gøtzsche PC, Ioannidis JP, Clarke M, Devereaux PJ, Kleijnen J, Moher D. The PRISMA statement for reporting systematic reviews and meta-analyses of studies that evaluate health care interventions: explanation and elaboration. PLoS Med, 2009, 6(7): e1000100.

267. Moher D, Shamseer L, Clarke M, Ghersi D, Liberati A, Petticrew M, Shekelle P, Stewart LA, PRISMA-P Group. Preferred reporting items for systematic review and meta-analysis protocols (PRISMA-P) 2015 statement. Syst Rev, 2015, 4: 1.

268. Shamseer L, Moher D, Clarke M, Ghersi D, Liberati A, Petticrew M, Shekelle P, Stewart LA, Group P-P. Preferred reporting items for systematic review and meta-analysis protocols (PRISMA-P) 2015: elaboration and explanation. BMJ, 2015, 349: g7647.

269. Zorzela L, Loke YK, Ioannidis JP, Golder S, Santaguida P, Altman DG, Moher D, Vohra S. PRISMA harms checklist: improving harms reporting in systematic reviews. BMJ, 2016, DOI: http://dx.doi.org/10.1136/bmj.i157. http://www.bmj.com/content/352/bmj.i157.

270. Hammad TA, Neyarapally GA, Pinheiro SP, Iyasu S, Rochester G, Dal Pan G. Reporting of meta-analyses of randomized controlled trials with a focus on drug safety: an empirical assessment. Clin Trials, 2013, 10(3): 389-397.

271. Stone M, Laughren T, Jones ML, Levenson M, Holland PC, Hughes A, Hammad TA, Temple R, Rochester G. Risk of suicidality in clinical trials of antidepressants in adults: analysis of proprietary data submitted to US Food and Drug Administration. BMJ, 2009, 339: b2880.

272. Lang T, Secic M. Considering "prior probabilities:" reporting Bayesian statistical analyses. in How to Report Statistics in Medicine: Annotated Guidelines for Authors, Editors, and Reviewers. 1997, American College of Physicians: Philadelphia. 231-235.

273. BaSiS Group. Bayesian Standards in Science: Standards for Reporting of Bayesian Analyses in the Scientific Literature. 2001. http://www.stat.cmu.edu/bayesworkshop/2001/BaSis.html.

274. Sung L, Hayden J, Greenberg ML, Koren G, Feldman BM, Tomlinson GA. Seven items were identified for inclusion when reporting a Bayesian analysis of a clinical study. J Clin Epidemiol, 2005, 58(3): 261-268.

275. Spiegelhalter DJ, Abrams KR, Myles JP. Bayesian approaches to clinical trials and health-care evaluation. 2004: Wiley. com.

276. Herbst AL, Ulfelder H, Poskanzer DC. Adenocarcinoma of the vagina. Association of maternal stilbestrol therapy with tumor appearance in young women. N Engl J Med, 1971, 284(15): 878-881.

277. Crowe B, Xia HA, Nilsson ME, Shahin S, Wang WV, Jiang Q. The program safety analysis plan: An implementation guide. in Quantitative evaluation of safety in drug development: Design, analysis, and reporting, Q. Jiang and H.A. Xia, Editors. 2015, Chapman & Hall: London. 55-68.

278. Xia HA, Jiang Q. Statistical evaluation of drug safety data. Therapeutic Innovation and Regulatory Science, 2014, 48(1): 109-120.

279. Ioannidis JP. Why most published research findings are false. PLoS Med, 2005, 2(8): e124.

280. Nüesch F, Trelle S, Reichenbach S, Rutjes AW, Tschannen B, Altman DG, Egger M, Juni P. Small study effects in meta-analyses of osteoarthritis trials: meta-epidemiological study. BMJ, 2010, 341: c3515.

281. Moreno SG, Sutton AJ, Thompson JR, Ades AE, Abrams KR, Cooper NJ. A generalized weighting regression-derived meta-analysis estimator robust to small-study effects and heterogeneity. Stat Med, 2012, 31(14): 1407-1417.

282. Kirkham JJ, Altman DG, Williamson PR. Bias due to changes in specified outcomes during the systematic review process. PLoS One, 2010, 5(3): e9810.

283. Trikalinos TA, Churchill R, Ferri M, Leucht S, Tuunainen A, Wahlbeck K, Ioannidis JP, project E-P. Effect sizes in cumulative meta-analyses of mental health randomized trials evolved over time. J Clin Epidemiol, 2004, 57(11): 1124-1130.

284. CIOMS Working Group IX. Practical approaches to risk minimisation for medicinal products: Report of CIOMS Working Group IX. 2014, Geneva, Switzerland: Council for International Organizations of Medical Sciences (CIOMS).

285. European Medicines Agency. Guideline on good pharmacovigilance practices (GVP): Module VI — – Management and reporting of adverse reactions to medicinal products (Rev 1) [online]. 2014, 28. http://www.ema.europa.eu/docs/en_GB/document_library/Scientific_guideline/2014/09/WC500172402.pdf.

286. Rezaie A. Absolute Versus Relative Risk: Can We Persuaded by Information Framing? Asian J Epidemiol, 2012, 5: 62-65.

287. European Medicines Agency. Guideline on good pharmacovigilance practices (GVP). Module XV – Safety communication. 2012. http://www.ema.europa.eu/docs/en_GB/document_library/Scientific_guideline/2013/01/WC500137666.pdf.

288. Uppsala Monitoring Centre. Dialogue in pharmacovigilance. 2002.

289. Uppsala Monitoring Centre. Effective communication in pharmacovigilance: the Erice report., in International Conference on Developing Effective Communications in Pharmacovigilance. 1997, Uppsala Monitoring Centre: Erice, Sicily, Italy.

290. Pamer CA, Hammad TA, Wu YT, Kaplan S, Rochester G, Governale L, Mosholder AD. Changes in US antidepressant and antipsychotic prescription patterns during a period of FDA actions. Pharmacoepidemiol Drug Saf, 2010, 19(2): 158-174.

291. AHRQ Agency for Healthcare Research and Quality. Methods Guide for Effectiveness and Comparative Effectiveness Reviews. 2014. http://effectivehealthcare.ahrq.gov/ehc/products/60/318/CER-Methods-Guide-140109.pdf.

292. European Medicines Agency. Points to consider on application with 1. meta-analyses; 2. one pivotal study. 2001. http://www.ema.europa.eu/docs/en_GB/document_library/Scientific_guideline/2009/09/WC500003657.pdf.

293. Sadock BJ, Sadock VA, Ruiz P, Kaplan HI. Kaplan & Sadock's comprehensive textbook of psychiatry. 9th ed. 2009, Philadelphia: Wolters Kluwer Health/Lippincott Williams & Wilkins.

294. U.S. Food and Drug Administration. FDA briefing document for the December 13, 2007 Psychopharmacologic Drugs Advisory Committee meeting. 2007. http://www.fda.gov/ohrms/dockets/ac/06/briefing/2006-4272b1-index.htm.

295. Gart JL. Point and interval estimation of the common odds ratio in the combination of 2 × 2 tables with fixed marginals. Biometrika, 1970, 57: 471-475.

296. Leyland-Jones B, BEST Investigators and Study Group. Breast cancer trial with erythropoietin terminated unexpectedly. Lancet Oncol, 2003, 4(8): 459-460.

297. Bohlius J, Wilson J, Seidenfeld J, Piper M, Schwarzer G, Sandercock J, Trelle S, Weingart O, Bayliss S, Brunskill S, Djulbegovic B, Benett CL, Langensiepen S, Hyde C, Engert E. Erythropoietin or darbepoetin for patients with cancer. Cochrane Database Syst Rev, 2006(3): CD003407.

298. Bennett CL, Silver SM, Djulbegovic B, Samaras AT, Blau CA, Gleason KJ, Barnato SE, Elverman KM, Courtney DM, McKoy JM, Edwards BJ, Tigue CC, Raisch DW, Yarnold PR, Dorr DA, Kuzel TM, Tallman MS, Trifilio SM, West DP, Lai SY, Henke M. Venous thromboembolism and mortality associated with recombinant erythropoietin and darbepoetin administration for the treatment of cancer-associated anemia. JAMA, 2008, 299(8): 914-924.

299. Glaspy J, Crawford J, Vansteenkiste J, Henry D, Rao S, Bowers P, Berlin JA, Tomita D, Bridges K, Ludwig H. Erythropoiesis-stimulating agents in oncology: a study-level meta-analysis of survival and other safety outcomes. Br J Cancer, 2010, 102(2): 301-315.

300. Tonelli M, Hemmelgarn B, Reiman T, Manns B, Reaume MN, Lloyd A, Wiebe N, Klarenbach S. Benefits and harms of erythropoiesis-stimulating agents for anemia related to cancer: a meta-analysis. CMAJ, 2009, 180(11): E62-71.

301. Erratum J. Incorrect data in: Inhaled anticholinergics and risk of major adverse cardiovascular events in patients with chronic obstructive pulmonary disease: a systematic review and meta-analysis. JAMA, 2009, 301(12): 1227-1230.

302. Tashkin DP, Celli B, Senn S, Burkhart D, Kesten S, Menjoge S, Decramer M, Investigators US. A 4-year trial of tiotropium in chronic obstructive pulmonary disease. N Engl J Med, 2008, 359(15): 1543-1554.

303. U.S. Food and Drug Administration. Early communication about an ongoing safety review of tiotropium [marketed as Spiriva HandiHaler]. 2008. http://www.fda.gov/Drugs/DrugSafety/PostmarketDrugSafetyInformationforPatientsandProviders/DrugSafetyInformationforHeathcareProfessionals/ucm070651.htm.

304. Home PD, Pocock SJ, Beck-Nielsen H, Gomis R, Hanefeld M, Jones NP, Komajda M, McMurray JJ, RECORD Study Group. Rosiglitazone evaluated for cardiovascular outcomes–an interim analysis. N Engl J Med, 2007, 357(1): 28-38.

305. Böhning D, Mylona K, Kimber A. Meta-analysis of clinical trials with rare events. Biom J, 2015, 57(4): 633-648.

306. Nissen SE, Wolski K. Rosiglitazone revisited: an updated meta-analysis of risk for myocardial infarction and cardiovascular mortality. Arch Intern Med, 2010, 170(14): 1191-1201.

307. Rossouw JE, Anderson GL, Prentice RL, LaCroix AZ, Kooperberg C, Stefanick ML, Jackson RD, Beresford SA, Howard BV, Johnson KC, Kotchen JM, Ockene J, Writing Group for the Women's Health Initiative I. Risks and benefits of estrogen plus progestin in healthy postmenopausal women: principal results From the Women's Health Initiative randomized controlled trial. JAMA, 2002, 288(3): 321-333.